Professional Ethics *in* Midwifery Practice

Illysa R. Foster, MEd, CPM
Licensed Midwife
Sisters Midwifery, Inc.
Austin, Texas

Jon Lasser, PhD
Associate Professor
Texas State University–San Marcos
San Marcos, Texas

JONES AND BARTLETT PUBLISHERS
Sudbury, Massachusetts
BOSTON   TORONTO   LONDON   SINGAPORE

World Headquarters

Jones and Bartlett Publishers	Jones and Bartlett Publishers	Jones and Bartlett Publishers
40 Tall Pine Drive	Canada	International
Sudbury, MA 01776	6339 Ormindale Way	Barb House, Barb Mews
978-443-5000	Mississauga, Ontario L5V 1J2	London W6 7PA
info@jbpub.com	Canada	United Kingdom
www.jbpub.com		

Jones and Bartlett's books and products are available through most bookstores and online book-sellers. To contact Jones and Bartlett Publishers directly, call 800-832-0034, fax 978-443-8000, or visit our website at www.jbpub.com.

Substantial discounts on bulk quantities of Jones and Bartlett's publications are available to corporations, professional associations, and other qualified organizations. For details and specific discount information, contact the special sales department at Jones and Bartlett via the above contact information or send an email to specialsales@jbpub.com.

The authors, editor, and publisher have made every effort to provide accurate information. However, they are not responsible for errors, omissions, or for any outcomes related to the use of the contents of this book and take no responsibility for the use of the products and procedures described. Treatments and side effects described in this book may not be applicable to all people; likewise, some people may require a dose or experience a side effect that is not described herein. Drugs and medical devices are discussed that may have limited availability controlled by the Food and Drug Administration (FDA) for use only in a research study or clinical trial. Research, clinical practice, and government regulations often change the accepted standard in this field. When consideration is being given to use of any drug in the clinical setting, the health care provider or reader is responsible for determining FDA status of the drug, reading the package insert, and reviewing prescribing information for the most up-to-date recommendations on dose, precautions, and contraindications, and determining the appropriate usage for the product. This is especially important in the case of drugs that are new or seldom used.

Production Credits

Publisher: Kevin Sullivan
Acquisitions Editor: Amy Sibley
Associate Editor: Patricia Donnelly
Editorial Assistant: Rachel Shuster
Associate Production Editor: Katie Spiegel
Marketing Manager: Rebecca Wasley
V.P., Manufacturing and Inventory Control:
    Therese Connell
Composition: Datastream Content Solutions, LLC
Cover Design: Scott Moden
Cover Image: © Robert George/Dreamstime.com
Printing and Binding: Malloy, Inc.
Cover Printing: Malloy, Inc.

Library of Congress Cataloging-in-Publication Data
Foster, Illysa R.
  Professional ethics in midwifery practice / Illysa R. Foster and Jon Lasser.
    p. ; cm.
  Includes bibliographical references and index.
  ISBN 978-0-7637-6880-5
1. Midwives—Professional ethics. I. Lasser, Jon, PhD. II. Title.
[DNLM: 1. Midwifery—ethics.   2. Ethics, Professional.   WQ 160 F755p 2011]
RG950.F64 2011
174.2'982—dc22

                                                    2009037357

6048

Printed in the United States of America
14 13 12 11 10   10 9 8 7 6 5 4 3 2 1

Dedication

For our daughters Jasmine and Sage, with love;
and for the midwives who have carried on the tradition and those who follow.

Contents

Preface

"The first step in the evolution of ethics is a sense of solidarity with other human beings" – Albert Schweitzer

Ethics is a broad field that has applications across disciplines and implications for nations, businesses, organizations, professionals, and individuals. It is a guiding set of principles that informs our actions, and a daily practice that is mitigated by contextual factors. Without ethics in our profession, midwives would be spiritually stagnant and metaphorically paralyzed by procedure, policy, and doctrine without thought for their implications. We would, in fact, be inhuman.

Our contribution to this field, the writing and publication of this book, is a small one. We are driven to contribute to midwifery in this way by our joint experiences. As a midwife, Illysa struggles with ethical decisions and seeks guidance from colleagues and the existing codes and literature. An applied ethics professor in the field of school psychology, Jon teaches students and other professionals about the practical side of ethics. Far from abstract, our effort here provides a midwifery-centered approach to ethics in practice. Our effort is not to be taken as the authority on midwifery ethics, but rather as a voice.

The presentation of chapters that you will read is a history of our journey into the rocky terrain of midwifery ethics. There are many sturdy structures and guideposts along the way, as well as deep crevasses that need bridging. We find wisdom in dissertations from Australia, ethical codes from Europe, a midwife from Mexico, and cross-disciplinary studies published in peer-reviewed journals in the United States. Along the way, a concept becomes clearer on the horizon: an ethical decision-making model of midwifery.

Rather than applying other models to a profession as vibrant and independent as midwifery, we nurture a homegrown model that is both academic and caring, professional and emotional, principle based and contextually embedded. It is intended for all midwives, regardless of practice setting or credential, because ethics is a necessary component of all midwifery service. It is also a place where midwives from all practice types come together. All midwives provide woman-centered care, and this book addresses the experiences of home-birth practice as well as hospital practice. Midwives are inclusive. We share an identity and we share in our ethical concerns.

The book is written with instruction in mind. Both authors have extensive experience teaching in higher education. We utilize case studies, as well as review and analysis of research findings, to engage critical thinking, a skill necessary for midwifery practitioners. Twelve chapters provide the instructor with a full semester of material, and we encourage ample use of independent research projects, group discussion, and debate alongside this book. These techniques will spark interest in midwifery ethics and, we hope, lead to further scholarly contributions.

Ultimately, that is our goal: to further the advancement of midwifery through ethics-based inquiry, publications, and professional development. We hope that ours is not the final word on ethics in the field, but rather a platform from which many voices will spring, speak, and build. We hope to improve the field of midwifery in a meaningful way by bringing ethics into the forefront of our collective endeavors: keeping our own home tidy can go far in making positive impressions on others.

Examination of existing ethical codes is a major component of the book. We find similarities and contrasts among codes to be an inspiration. We include nearly every aspect of the codes in the book and add other topics. These include multiple relationships, defining the client, and ethical decision making. The existing ethical codes are a tremendous source of well-conceived structures regarding ethics.

The Midwives Model of Care is evident in all components of the ethics presented in this book because it best represents the work we do. The heart of our work is partnership with women and their families and support for natural birth, along with skills and competence. Our care is individualized, and we try to honor this in each ethical consideration that we cover in this book. Biomedical ethical theories can be helpful, but also hindering, for midwives who work in relationship with others.

We believe that ethical standards have a central role in midwifery. We trust women and midwives, but we must hold one another and our profession to the highest ethical standards because the work we do and the profession we hold dearly deserve it. Although midwifery may very well be the oldest profession, modern professional midwifery is in its infancy. Consequently, midwives must develop strong professional standards so that we can maintain autonomy and continue practicing midwifery the way we want. The voices of traditional midwives who continued the art of midwifery from the dawn of time are still among us, but we have entered the era of professionalism; from the trails of the Frontier Nursing Service and the halls of Congress, we have defined ourselves as professional midwives in the United States. It is imperative that we adopt and adhere to ethical standards.

We do not advocate for blind allegiance to codes of ethics, nor do we view the world in stark black and white. Ethical decisions are enveloped in complex contextual factors that must be considered. The challenge of ethical practice is to understand both code and context, standard and setting, client and culture. We also recognize that, more often than not, navigating these complexities is made easier with the help of colleagues, consultation with experts, and the utilization of texts in ethics.

Ethics is a process, an ongoing growth-oriented ebb and flow. We use the phrase "doing ethics" at the end of the text to reflect this perspective. The term *ethics* is akin to the term *midwifery*, both noun and verb. By practicing midwifery, you become a midwife. By practicing ethics, you become an ethical midwife. You may not be the most highly skilled midwife when you graduate, and we do not expect a reading of our book to make each student an ethicist. Rather, we hope that you will learn to think ethically, with a vocabulary of constructs that are presented here as your cognitive tool set. We also hope that you enjoy the journey, as we have.

Illysa R. Foster, MEd, CPM
Jon Lasser, PhD

Acknowledgments

Embarking on the daunting task of writing our first book, we were aware that we would require much assistance. However, we were humbled by the number of kind and generous individuals willing to offer their time, expertise, and skills in helping us with the process. Special thanks go to Rachel Shuster at Jones and Bartlett for answering countless questions by email (usually on the same day they were sent) and providing guidance about the publishing process to novices. Thanks also to Amy Sibley, Katie Spiegel, and Rebecca Wasley at Jones and Bartlett for their assistance. We acknowledge and thank Nadine Stellavato Brown at Lost Luggage, who produced a beautiful rendering of our model that captured the idea in visual form. Nick Kotz and Zac Rolnik provided helpful advice about the publishing business. Many of the sources used in the book were gathered tirelessly by the incomparable James Diep. James, along with Elizabeth Young and Patricia Petmecky, helped us check each chapter for consistency, references, and so forth. We also wish to thank the many midwives who shared case examples, provided feedback on our model, and supported us in writing this book. In particular, we wish to recognize Christy Tashjian, Mary Barnett, Alison Bastien, MariMikel Penn, Gera Simkins, Sister Angela Murdaugh, Laurie Fremgen, Becca Price, and Anne Frye.

We thank the following organizations for providing permission to reproduce their ethical codes and other documents: the Midwives Alliance of North America, the American College of Nurse-Midwives, the International Confederation of Midwives, the National Association of Certified Professional Midwives, the Nursing and Midwifery Council, and the North American Registry of Midwives.

Finally, this book would not be possible without the love, support, and patience of our daughters, Jasmine and Sage. Our maternal grandmothers, Ramona Clements and Sarah Yarrin, with unwavering and exaggerated confidence in our abilities, helped through their constant belief in us. Don Foster, Carmen Clements, Ellen Lasser, Tommy Kaye, and Jon Lasser Sr. provided parental guidance and support.

CHAPTER 1

Why Ethics for Midwives?

Students of midwifery, nursing, psychology, social work, medicine, and other helping professions are often required to take coursework in the area of ethics. To many, the field of ethics may seem irrelevant, abstract, or esoteric. Ethics is often associated with philosophy or religion and therefore presumed to be unrelated to professional training. Typically, students are excited about developing the practical skills of midwifery, so it is understandable that some may find theoretical or philosophical approaches less appealing. It is our hope that this book will persuade you that ethics is not only relevant to the training of professional midwives, but also that it is essential and practical.

For the most part, this book does *not* utilize a philosophical/religious orientation to ethics for midwives. Rather, we have written this text as a midwife's resource for applied professional ethics, which enables us to think about, understand, and address real professional problems faced by practicing midwives through the lens of ethical principles, rules, and codes (Nash, 2002). Our goal is to make your study of ethics relevant to your training and work rather than abstract and detached. To this end, we bring core ethical issues to life with vivid case examples that midwives are likely to encounter in daily practice.

In this introduction, we identify several reasons why ethics are important for midwifery, address some background concerns regarding applied professional ethics, and discuss some broad ethical frameworks. Additionally, we place ethics for midwives in the larger context of the Midwives Model of Care (MMOC) (Rothman, 1979). Finally, we conclude this chapter with an overview of the book and how to best use it.

THE IMPORTANCE OF ETHICS

There are numerous reasons midwives are and should be concerned with professional ethics, but all of those reasons can be condensed into one general statement: ethics in midwifery is good for clients, midwives, and the profession. Our ethical guidelines serve to protect the interests of all parties and provide guidance through difficult decision-making processes. We should therefore spend some time exploring the ways in which applied professional ethics serve these various stakeholders.

Ethics Encourage Self-Regulation

A primary and critical role of applied professional ethics is self-regulation. Professional midwives know that the development of ethical codes and guidelines communicates clearly to governmental regulatory agencies that midwives have the capacity to regulate themselves. In the absence of professional ethics, the state often intervenes to regulate. Self-regulation is preferred because no one knows a profession better than its members. Historically, physicians' professional organizations such as the American Medical Association (AMA) and the American College of Obstetricians and Gynecologists (ACOG) have tried, through political efforts, to regulate and limit the practice of midwives (ACOG, 2008a; AMA, 2008; Rooks, 1999a). Thus, the development of ethical standards for midwives can be seen as a clear effort to maintain internal regulation and avoid external regulation. Internal regulation is always preferred, and it has the potential to limit and shape external regulation. For example, with licensure, states are in the position to shape midwifery practice. When midwives regulate themselves, governing bodies are less likely to interfere with and restrict practice.

Ethics Foster Professional Identity

Professions are groups of individuals who share a common set of knowledge and skills with specialized training and provide services to the public (Beauchamp & Childress, 2009). When a field develops a set of shared beliefs about ethical practice, professional identity grows and solidifies. This is particularly important in midwifery, because there is a need to differentiate what midwives do from other related fields. Consumers may question the differences among midwives, doulas, obstetricians, and other care providers associated with birth. By developing a profession-specific set of ethical guidelines, midwives communicate a unique role and function. This process informs consumers, lawmakers, primary care physicians, and the public that midwifery has an identity that is distinct from, yet related to, other birth professionals. This identity formation is critical not only for differentiating midwives from nonmidwives but also for clarifying similarities and differences among midwives (e.g., direct-entry midwives vs. nurse–midwives). Thus, our ethical codes serve as an important way of defining ourselves and communicating who we are in relation to others.

Ethics Protect Midwives and Clients

Professional ethics function as a protective measure for consumers and care providers. Ethics are proactive signposts that help us make decisions about how we behave toward others. For example, our ethics direct us to respect the dignity of our clients and honor their autonomy. In this regard, professional ethics inform decisions about how we treat others before we interact with them. Moreover, our clients expect ethical standards from midwifery. Thompson (2007) states, "[T]he primary reason for being ethical/professional is based on the mandate from society to any professional group licensed to practice their profession" (p. 279). Ethical conduct flows directly from our codes and values.

The proactive nature of ethics gives us the opportunity to anticipate potential conflicts and plan for optimal outcomes. Consider the value midwives place on fairness and integrity in relationships to others (Midwives Alliance of North America, 1997). Awareness of this value prepares midwives for the resolution of potential conflicts, such as a client's difficulty paying for services. The value of maintaining integrity guides the midwife toward a resolution that preserves the professional-client relationship. Conflict resolution that respects and maintains good midwife-client relations serves to protect both midwives and clients. Although proactive ethics are ideal, professional ethics typically evolve in a reactive manner.

Professional ethics often emerge as a response to an observed pattern of problems. As a profession grows and develops, a critical mass of concerns or complaints spurs the development of an ethical guideline to address the pattern. This reactive approach is common across professions and is largely caused by the challenges of anticipating tomorrow's ethical dilemmas. Changes in technology, law, and culture are hard to predict and may have significant bearings on ethical decision making. Nevertheless, midwives should strive to develop proactive ethics, understanding that a reactive approach may sometimes be necessary.

Ethical protections for consumers and professionals have a secondary benefit: greater confidence in the profession. One of the reasons that any profession develops an ethical code or set of ethical guidelines and principles is to promote public confidence in the profession. The field of sociology has given considerable attention to the importance of public confidence and suggests that the public's perception of a profession's trustworthiness is essential for the establishment of "professional status" (Pescosolido, Tuch, & Martin, 2001). The American College of Nurse-Midwives (ACNM) states in its Code of Ethics (2008) that "midwives support and maintain the integrity of the profession of midwifery and thus contribute to a profession worthy of being considered by society as a public good" (p. 2).

Consider a profession that you do not trust. Are you skeptical about their services? Do you feel uncomfortable in your working relationships with them? Mistrust may be related to a sense that the profession lacks ethical standards and conduct. However, professions that have clear ethical guidelines, communicate those guidelines to consumers, and strive to maintain ethical conduct foster trust, confidence, and respect from the public.

Ethical guidelines for midwives play a critical role in the promotion of public confidence. The general public and other healthcare professionals have a more favorable opinion of midwifery when they understand that midwives take ethics seriously, have invested energy in the development of ethical guidelines, and work toward maintaining ethical conduct. In this regard, the benefits of applied professional ethics (e.g., protection of consumers and midwives, professional identity, and differentiation) are interrelated.

Ethics Signal Professional Maturity

The growth, development, and maturation of a profession can be compared to the developmental stages of an organism. Just as crawling and babbling represent developmental milestones in infancy, so too a profession's maturity is marked by significant events. One indicator of a profession's maturity is the development of ethical codes, guidelines, and conduct.

Ethical codes of conduct reflect a level of professionalism that midwives have long sought to achieve. Even as midwifery in the United States has developed from two separate identities, nurse–midwives and direct-entry midwives, a shared identity as "midwife" has prevailed, bringing the ACNM and the Midwives Alliance of North America (MANA) perhaps closer than ever before in holding a space for midwifery as an important component of maternity care. Because ethics is a shared concern among midwives, it is common ground for all midwives to distinguish themselves from other health and human service professions.

Both MANA and ACNM have struggled to be recognized as professional maternity care providers by physicians and governing bodies (Rooks, 1999a). These efforts to assert professional identity have played out at the local, state, and national levels in areas of licensure, prescription privileges, physician supervision, and others. Today, physicians are still actively seeking limitations on midwives' rights to practice independently and out of the hospital. At times, these struggles have led to divisive debates between direct-entry midwives and nurse–midwives.

The effort to defend midwifery has fueled a long history of splits between professional organizations. Often, divisions between ACNM and MANA revolve around issues of professionalism, the most divisive involving educational requirements and direct-entry training. With the direct-entry route now espoused by ACNM in the form of the certified midwife (CM), and MANA supporting accreditation for midwifery training programs through the Midwifery Education Accreditation Council (MEAC) and a professional certification (Certified Professional Midwife), it is evident that even these deepest of divisions are narrowing. In the United States, nurse–midwives and direct-entry midwives must overcome differences and unify as "midwives" in order for midwifery to flourish (Davis-Floyd & Johnson, 2006).

Shared ethical guidelines increase cohesiveness among midwives, strengthening the identity of "midwife" across differences in training, practice site, income, and clientele, because ethics apply across these variables. Whether you are serving low-income immigrant women in a Southwest border-town birth center or upper middle class women in a maternity hospital in New England, ethical conduct applies. At the same time, ethics are informed by the specific contextual and individual factors that exist in a setting and clinician relationship. Ethics are essential to the application of the MMOC.

Limitations of Ethical Codes

We must also recognize that although ethical codes serve many purposes, there are significant limitations to published ethical guidelines. The code of ethics of the International Confederation of Midwives (ICM, 1999) provides useful commentary about what ethical codes *do not* do. Ethical codes in and of themselves cannot guarantee ethical behavior or best practices. As an articulation of values and standards, a code cannot actually regulate behavior, nor can it completely provide midwives with the guidance they seek when faced with ethical dilemmas. Perhaps most important, ICM poignantly states that "a code cannot remove from midwives the responsibility and pain of living and acting, at times, in situations of ambiguity or 'not knowing', of having no in-built guarantees about what, in a given case, constitutes 'right action'" (p. 7). In this regard, we are reminded that codes serve as guidelines that may assist midwives with the hard work of serving women and families in complex, real-world situations.

ETHICS: AN OVERVIEW

Searching for a definition of *ethics* or the related term *morality* can lead to considerable frustration, as these words have multiple meanings depending on context and usage. A brief review of writings on the subjects of ethics and morals suggests that many authors (e.g., Frankena, 1973; Nash, 2002) use the terms interchangeably, begging the question "What's the difference?" This section discusses the differences between morals and ethics, identifies some problems with ethical systems, and addresses the need for applied professional ethics.

Before we can introduce ethics, we first need to address morals. *Morality* generally refers to standards of behavior or conduct, whereas *ethics* is often considered the branch of philosophy that studies moral systems. Our morals provide us with general guidelines regarding our relationships with others, such as "treat others with dignity and respect." A moral dilemma arises when we realize that we are faced with a conflict involving our treatment of others. Such conflicts may occur when our effort to uphold one moral standard conflicts with another moral standard (type I dilemmas). Alternatively, a moral dilemma may arise in trying to uphold one moral principle for one person that would result in violating the same principle for another person (type II dilemmas) (Frankena, 1973).

To illustrate type I dilemmas, we explore the conflict between providing appropriate care and maintaining client autonomy. Consider this example: A client has tested positive for group B strep, and the midwife recommends the use of antibiotics during labor. However, the client communicates that she does not want to receive antibiotics. Should the midwife respect the client's autonomy at the expense of the standard of care?

This example demonstrates how morals can be in conflict with one another. We are frequently faced with such situations in our personal and professional lives and often seek guidance from friends, colleagues, and advisors. Although this guidance may be helpful, it may also complicate matters. The midwife consulting with colleagues is likely to receive conflicting suggestions. What is needed is a system for resolving these moral dilemmas. We will address this after we consider an example that illustrates type II dilemmas.

American philosopher Robert Kane (1994), building on the work of Immanuel Kant, proposed a moral framework called the Ends Principle: to "treat every person as an end and not as a means (to your or someone else's ends) whenever possible" (p. 26). This suggests that we should respect the values of others, let them pursue their goals and desires, and avoid imposing our values and desires on them. In doing so, we refrain from forcing others to do things against their will. This seems clear enough, but we don't have to look far for examples of moral dilemmas stemming directly from this one principle.

Suppose that a midwife and physician are co-managing the care of a client, and the physician is intervening in a way that is not desired by the client. According to the Ends Principle, the midwife should attempt to treat the physician and client in a way that permits each to pursue their individual goals. However, allowing the physician to pursue his goals interferes with the client's goals. Kane (1994) would argue that the physician has stepped outside the "moral sphere" by overriding the client's goals and, in doing so, has lost his right to pursue his goals. In other words, the Ends Principle has a built-in caveat: under most circumstances, we allow everyone to purse their ends, but there may be situations in which our efforts to allow one party to pursue his or her goals results in another party not being able to pursue his or her goals.

Thompson (2007) provides a clear application of the Ends Principle to the practice of midwifery: "Simply put, midwives should not use the women they care for to meet their own needs for nurturing, parenting, maintaining control, or the like. Midwives must view women and their health needs as ends in themselves, worthy of respect and caring" (p. 283). We believe that midwives may reap great personal benefit from serving women, and that such gains should not be considered unethical. Rather, the joy, pleasure, and financial compensation are legitimately earned benefits. The key point is that we do not regard our clients as means to our ends, but rather as ends in themselves.

Ethical dilemmas are not limited to ends and means. We also experience challenges when our thoughts and feelings about morals differ from those of others, or when our priorities regarding moral obligations do not align with those of others. For example, in an emergency situation in which both the mother's and baby's life are in jeopardy, midwives, other birth attendants, and family members may have conflicting notions of moral obligations. Such conflicts raise questions about the possibility of applying absolute standards across settings.

These examples challenge us to think about the limitations of moral principles and encourage us to seek greater clarity and guidance. We need a way to think about and process moral decisions that is grounded and useful. Ethics helps us identify the best decision by applying systematic thought to these dilemmas.

A basic definition of ethics serves as a useful starting point for our discussion. Beauchamp and Childress (2009) describe ethics as "a generic term covering several different ways of examining and understanding the moral life" (p. 1). Ethics can also be understood as the "search for clarity and cogency in one's beliefs about the nature of the good life and right conduct" (Munitz, 1958, p. 2). Embedded in this definition is an assumption that bad behavior exists, for if it did not we would not need to spend time thinking about "right conduct." The fact of the matter is that from time to time we have doubts about the correctness of our own behavior and the behavior of others. We have a number of standards by which behaviors are judged (e.g., religion, law, tradition), but these standards are frequently called into question. Consider the prohibition against killing, which is found in most religions and laws. Are we willing to make exceptions to this prohibition? Is killing acceptable as a means of self-defense, for criminal punishment, in war, or for euthanasia? Such doubts regarding the applicability of ethical standards drive the study of ethics. We now turn our attention to the limitations of commonsense ethics, ethical relativism, and the objectivity of Western ethics.

A conventional or "commonsense" approach to ethics is often used as a guiding principle. For example, notions of justice, fairness, and equality are often invoked as standards by which we should live our lives. The primary problems with this approach, colorfully illustrated in Plato's *Republic*, concern the vague, inflexible, and inconsistent ways in which such standards are applied (Munitz, 1958). Rigid adherence to equality (in the sense of everyone getting the same treatment) does not permit the flexibility needed when we recognize that as individuals we have unique needs. For example, one might argue that giving everyone identical food rations would exemplify fair, just, and equitable distribution of resources, yet as individuals we have different dietary needs.

Another problem with ethical standards concerns *relativism*, or the recognition that there are diverse belief systems and no rational way of determining which belief system is the best or correct one (Kane, 1994; Munitz, 1958). Many contemporary social issues are contested because various belief systems are in conflict. Consider the movement to legalize the use of marijuana. One side argues that marijuana should not be legal and that its use is basically wrong, whereas the other side favors legalization and does not view the use of marijuana as unethical. Regardless of the position taken, one must recognize that the task of identifying one "correct" or "right" belief is futile, for there is no rational basis for doing so. This problem of relativism should not be taken lightly, because it has profound implications for how we treat one another in a pluralistic society.

Some scholars in nursing have highlighted the shortcomings of conventional approaches to ethics and have promoted a "context-sensitive approach" (Lützén, 1997, p. 218). This perspective argues that a traditional, Western approach to ethics fails to meet the demands of daily practice. This may in part be due to the reliance of traditional ethics on objectivity and impartiality, whereas the real-world experiences of daily practice involve subjectivity and partiality. Advances in medical technology and greater attention to issues of diversity and multiculturalism also test the limits of traditional ethical paradigms.

Broad Ethical Principles

Beauchamp and Childress (2009) have identified basic principles of common morality that serve as a framework for their work on biomedical ethics. Each element of our professional ethical codes can be linked to one or more of these broad principles. Therefore, the following four principles provide a guide for ethical practice (pp. 12–13):

1. *Respect for autonomy* (a norm of respecting and supporting autonomous decisions)
2. *Nonmaleficence* (a norm of avoiding the causation of harm)
3. *Beneficence* (a group of norms pertaining to relieving, lessening, or preventing harm and providing benefits and balancing benefits against risks and costs)
4. *Justice* (a group of norms for fairly distributing benefits, risks, and costs)

These four principles will be referenced throughout the book so that readers will have an explicit connection between professional ethical codes and the overarching morals from which they were derived. In daily practice, our challenge is not only to address these principles but also to balance the demands of each of them. What follows is a brief explanation of each principle.

Respect for Autonomy

Individuals have certain rights that should be acknowledged and supported, including the "right to hold views, to make choices, and to take actions based on their personal values and beliefs" (Beauchamp & Childress, 2009, p. 103). This means that we allow and encourage others to make decisions for themselves. Naturally, this becomes very complicated when we have to determine who receives the designation of an "autonomous agent" (and who does not). Nevertheless, we acknowledge that everyone has worth and should be allowed to pursue his or her hopes, dreams, and desires so long as they don't interfere with others. Recognizing and encouraging client autonomy stems from a more general respect for the dignity of others (Jacob & Hartshorne, 2003).

Nonmaleficence

Many readers are familiar with the idea of nonmaleficence, if not the word, because it is commonly expressed with the phrase "Above all [or first] do no harm" (Beauchamp & Childress, 2009, p. 149). From this seemingly simple principle come some basic ideas: do not kill, do not cause pain or suffering, and so on. A deeper exploration of this principle would require an expanded definition of harm, consideration of unintentional harm (due perhaps to neglect), the distinction between killing and letting die, and so forth. For our purposes, we will take a simplified approach by stating that one does not intentionally cause harm and also takes steps to prevent harm. This is a moral obligation that should be applied in all cases. Sometimes discussions of biomedical ethical principles collapse nonmaleficence and beneficence into one principle, but we feel that they are distinct.

Beneficence

The moral obligation to act for the benefit of others is known as beneficence. The notion of obligation complicates this principle, because some theorists argue that acts of beneficence are not required in all situations (Beauchamp & Childress, 2009). We should also differentiate nonmaleficence and beneficence, because the two terms are related. As we mentioned earlier, nonmaleficence is an obligation to do no harm. Conversely, beneficence is an action intended to promote some benefit to others. Whereas we are always obligated to do no harm, we may not always be obligated to act beneficently, particularly toward those with whom we have no special relationship (Beauchamp & Childress, 2009).

Justice

Of the four broad ethical principles described, justice may be the most complex. Multiple definitions and meanings of justice exist, as well as competing theories. For midwives, concerns about justice are related to inequalities in access to health care, fairness, opportunity, and unjust discrimination. Consequently, the concept of justice is applied to issues of diversity, equity, and egalitarian distribution of resources (Beauchamp & Childress, 2009). We limit our discussion of justice here and refer readers to Chapter 10, in which we discuss justice in greater detail.

APPLIED PROFESSIONAL ETHICS

Ethics is a broad field that includes a variety of theories and philosophical orientations. The preceding overview of ethics provides a general orientation and highlights the limitations of widely used ethical systems. This background encourages us to seek better ways of addressing ethical thinking in professional midwifery. Because this book was written to address ethics for midwives, we take a more specific approach. When dealing with the codes of conduct for a profession, we typically speak of *applied professional ethics*, or the implementation of ethical guidelines in real-world work situations. Therefore, this book addresses the ways in which *midwives* use ethical thinking to make the best professional decisions. Ethics for midwives can best be understood in the context of the MMOC.

The Midwives Model of Care

The MMOC is an independent model that both describes and guides midwives in providing care to women in the childbearing year. This model was first described by Rothman in 1979 as a contrast to the medical model of care for maternity patients. Since then, midwives have adopted an edited version of the definition.

The Midwives Model of Care™ is based on the fact that pregnancy and birth are normal life events. The Midwives Model of Care includes:

- monitoring the physical, psychological and social well-being of the mother throughout the childbearing cycle;
- providing the mother with individualized education, counseling, and prenatal care, continuous hands-on assistance during labor and delivery, and postpartum support;
- minimizing technological interventions and;
- identifying and referring women who require obstetrical attention.

The application of this model has been proven to reduce the incidence of birth injury, trauma, and cesarean section. (MANA, 2008, para. 13).

The MMOC is woman-centered, and women share in making decisions about their maternity care. Midwives are interested in the opinions, knowledge, concerns, and goals of the women and families that they serve (Rooks, 1999b). Midwives typically provide care for the mother-baby unit throughout pregnancy, birth, and the postpartum/newborn periods, developing enduring bonds with women and their families. Rooks elaborates:

In addition, the baby is not the only important outcome of the pregnancy. Pregnancy, especially every first pregnancy, is a critical developmental process for a woman. Pregnancy results in a *mother* as well as a baby. It is important that the woman's transition into motherhood is a positive experience, that she and all members of her family make emotionally healthy adjustments to each pregnancy and birth, and that she has the means to acquire the necessary information, skills, support, and self-confidence needed to successfully assume the roles and responsibilities of motherhood. Breastfeeding and mothercraft are part of the focus of midwifery. (Rooks, 1999b, p. 373)

In contrast to this model, Robbie Davis-Floyd describes the "technocratic model" of birth employed by obstetricians in the United States. Historically linked to the "body-as-machine" theories of Enlightenment philosophers, the technocratic model views women as inherently deviant and inferior to the male ideal. As such, the female body in the act of giving birth is dysfunctional, requiring a properly trained mechanic and technological tools. A dualistic philosophy is applied to the mother-baby unit, in effect separating the two even before birth. The entire birth procedure is conceptualized as an assembly-line model, whereby the "perfect baby" is the desired product, the doctor is the producer, and the new mother is a by-product. This is illustrated in ritual form in hospital births, beginning with the hospital gown upon admittance and ending with maternal-infant separation in the nursery. Davis-Floyd (1993, 2004) explains the use of such rituals as fulfilling a need to provide a sense of control over a natural process that is often unpredictable.

Whereas the technocratic model influences the code of ethics for obstetrician-gynecologists, midwifery ethics reflect the MMOC. In reading the ACOG Code of Professional Ethics, one can detect concern for overuse of medical devices and treatments in its warning against both undue influence by pharmaceutical companies and unwarranted medical procedures (ACOG, 2008b). Ethical guidelines assist physicians in practicing medicine (i.e., in implementing the medical model). Ethics are grounded in background beliefs, or a previous set of philosophical and metaphysical underpinnings (Nash, 2002). Physicians and midwives, as healthcare professionals caring for women, certainly share many background beliefs. "We study ethics because we are professionals who make decisions with and for others, and we need to understand what constitutes a good or correct decision for everyone involved" (Thompson, 2007, p. 289). Midwives largely identify with ACOG's ethical code as it applies to issues of personal privacy, informed consent, and scope of practice. Yet, contrasting belief systems about pregnancy and birth, as illustrated by Rothman and Davis-Floyd, separately inform ethics in these two fields. Conversely, ethical principles are reflected in the MMOC. The relationship between ethics and model of care is reciprocal. Together, midwifery ethics and the Midwives Model of Care influence the individual midwife's ethical decision making and practice.

OVERVIEW OF THIS BOOK

We have organized this book to facilitate your study of ethics in midwifery. The chapters are sequenced such that broad, general principles precede specific concepts so that you will have sufficient prior knowledge. This introductory chapter serves as a starting point for what we hope will be a stimulating and engaging exploration of applied professional ethics in midwifery. This book should ideally be used as a text for coursework in professional midwifery, either in conjunction with a course specifically dealing with ethics or a more general course on professional issues in midwifery, as well as a reference for practicing midwives.

We must also consider the relationships between ethical and legal concerns. The legal status of an act does not necessarily make it ethical. For example, a direct-entry midwife providing services in a state that prohibits midwifery may be acting ethically but illegally. Similarly, that which is legal may also be unethical. This book primarily addresses ethical concerns in midwifery and limits discussion of legal issues to those that intersect with midwifery. Therefore, this book should not be considered a comprehensive account of legal issues. State laws governing the practice of midwifery vary greatly, making state midwifery associations the best source for the current laws pertaining to midwives in your state. However, this book does address some of the larger issues related to the intersection of ethics and law that impact the practice of professional midwifery across the United States.

To get the most out of this text, we recommend reading it in the sequence in which it is presented. Although some chapters can serve as standalone readings, we have developed the book such that chapters build on one another and ultimately function as a whole that is greater than the sum of its parts.

We also firmly believe that knowledge is socially constructed and that progress is made when we collaborate and develop shared understanding. To this end, we hope that midwives and students of midwifery will read and discuss the book, and in particular the case examples, to promote debate, consensus, and forward-evolving professional ethics. The case studies and questions that follow them are well suited for homework assignments or group discussion starting points, or both.

Chapter 2 provides a discussion of the existing ethical codes, standards, and value statements that have been produced by national and international midwifery organizations (e.g., ICM, ACNM, MANA, National Association of Certified Professional Midwives). Following a review of these documents, we raise some questions about the profession's needs and how the profession can be served through improvements to the existing codes and standards. Some of these codes have been reproduced in the appendices of this text.

The remaining chapters cover specific ethical issues in professional midwifery, illustrated with case examples. Chapter 3 introduces the concepts of privacy and confidentiality in general and then more specifically as applied to the practice of professional midwifery in a wide range of situations (e.g., records, communication with clients, peer review). Informed consent is the subject of Chapter 4 and is framed as an ongoing process rather than a discrete event. Chapter 5 raises a fundamental yet often overlooked question: Who is the client? Chapter 6 concerns the ethical issues that arise from multiple relationships, and Chapter 7 discusses midwives' scope of practice and limits of competency. Chapter 8 concerns the ethical issues that arise when working with colleagues and other professionals. Client noncompliance and termination of care are reviewed in Chapter 9. In Chapter 10 we explore ethics in the context of diversity, justice, and equity. Chapter 11 focuses on ways to address ethical concerns when they arise, and in Chapter 12 we propose a new model of ethics for professional midwifery that reflects both principle-based ethics and situational-based concerns within the context of the midwife-client relationship.

Studying ethics will strengthen midwifery as a profession, promote public confidence in midwives, and protect clients, colleagues, and others from harm. Ultimately, ethics in midwifery helps us work in a context of care, respect, and justice. We recognize that ethical dilemmas are not easily resolved, but we hope that a working knowledge of ethical problems, standards, and models will help midwives make difficult decisions with good outcomes.

REFERENCES

American College of Nurse-Midwives (ACNM). (2008). *American College of Nurse-Midwives code of ethics with explanatory statements*. Silver Spring, MD: Author.

American College of Obstetricians and Gynecologists (ACOG). (2008a). *ACOG statement on home births*. Retrieved July 5, 2008, from http://www.acog.org/from_home/publications/press_releases/nr02-06-08-2.cfm

American College of Obstetricians and Gynecologists (ACOG). (2008b). *Code of professional ethics of the American College of Obstetricians and Gynecologists*. Retrieved July 5, 2008, from http://acog.org/from_home/publications/ethics

American Medical Association (AMA). (2008). *House of Delegates resolution 204*. Retrieved July 5, 2008, from http://www.ama-assn.org/ama/pub/category/18587.html

Beauchamp, T. L., & Childress, J. F. (2009). *Principles of biomedical ethics* (6th ed.). New York: Oxford University Press.

Davis-Floyd, R. E. (1993). The technocratic model of birth. In S. Tower Hollis, L. Pershing, & M. J. Young (Eds.), *Feminist theory and the study of folklore* (pp. 297–326). Champaign, IL: University of Illinois Press.

Davis-Floyd, R. E. (2004). *Birth as an American rite of passage*. Berkeley, CA: University of California Press.

Davis-Floyd, R. E., & Johnson, C.B. (2006). *Mainstreaming midwives: The politics of change*. New York: Routledge.

Frankena, W. K. (1973). *Ethics* (2nd ed.). Englewood Cliffs, NJ: Prentice-Hall.

International Confederation of Midwives (ICM). (1999). *ICM international code of ethics for midwives*. Retrieved November 3, 2008, from http://www.internationalmidwives.org/Documentation/Coredocuments/tabid/322/Default.aspx

Jacob, S., & Hartshorne, T. S. (2003). *Ethics and law for school psychologists*. Hoboken, NJ: Wiley.

Kane, R. (1994). *Through the moral maze: Searching for absolute values in a pluralistic world*. New York: Paragon House.

Lützén, K. (1997). Nursing ethics into the next millennium: A context-sensitive approach for nursing ethics. *Nursing Ethics, 4*(3), 218–226.

Midwives Alliance of North America (MANA). (1997). *Statement of values and ethics*. Washington, DC: Author.

Midwives Alliance of North America (MANA). (2008). *Definitions*. Retrieved September 16, 2009, from http://mana.org/definitions.html

Munitz, M. K. (1958). *A modern introduction to ethics: Readings from classical and contemporary sources*. Glencoe, IL: The Free Press.

Nash, R. J. (2002). *"Real world" ethics: Frameworks for educators and human service professionals*. New York: Teachers College Press.

Pescosolido, B. A., Tuch, S. A., & Martin, J. K. (2001). The profession of medicine and the public: Examining Americans' changing confidence in physician authority from the beginning of the 'health care crisis' to the era of health care reform. *Journal of Health and Social Behavior, 42*(1), 1–16.

Rooks, J. P. (1999a). *Midwifery and childbirth in America*. Philadelphia: Temple University Press.

Rooks, J. P. (1999b). The midwifery model of care. *Journal of Nurse-Midwifery, 44*(4), 370–374.

Rothman, B. K. (1979). *Two models in maternity care: Defining and negotiating reality*. New York: New York University Press.

Thompson, J. E. (2007). Professional ethics. In L. A. Ament (Ed.), *Professional issues in midwifery* (pp. 277–300). Sudbury, MA: Jones and Bartlett.

CHAPTER 2

Existing Ethical Codes, Guidelines, and Value Statements

BEFORE THE PUBLISHED DOCUMENTS

Midwifery has been called the world's oldest profession, although commentators have pointed out the fact that others lay claim to the title as well (Lopez Lysne, 2006). As mentioned in the previous chapter, the development of formal ethical codes represents professional maturity, a developmental milestone for the field. Given the deep and rich history of midwifery relative to "young" professions such as psychology and genetics, why have midwives only recently developed formal ethical codes and guidelines?

Although the documentation may be scant, we suspect that midwives worldwide have always operated under some ethical guidelines. Most likely, ethics were handed down in an oral tradition and were community specific. Imagine living in a small, rural village, isolated from the rest of the world. As the village midwife, you have a relationship with every member of the community and a shared sense of how you should treat mothers, fathers, elders, and children. Moreover, you also have a clear understanding of the consequences associated with various transgressions. Your behavior may not be under the scrutiny of a licensing board or professional organization, but it is certainly evaluated by your sisters, neighbors, parents, children, and other villagers.

If an oral tradition of ethics worked for so long, why in recent times have we moved to published codes of ethics, licensure and certification, legal parameters on practice, and all that comes with these changes? There may be many causes, among them the shift from rural to urban societies, the rise in litigation, increased specialization in health care, the pressures placed on midwifery by physicians, and the need for midwifery to define and differentiate itself from other professions. In this context, midwifery's development of documented ethical codes and guidelines represents a response to changing times and a culture of regulation.

We suspect that midwifery has also only recently developed ethical codes because, in many respects, the modern midwife is on the fringe. She has chosen an alternative path, rejecting a medical model of birth in favor of the Midwives Model of Care (MMOC) (Rothman, 1979). The establishment has also marginalized the midwife, marking her as a pariah of pregnancy. So perhaps the social positioning of midwifery has also contributed to the wide gap between the profession's origins and its development of published codes.

We are reminded that many traditional midwives, mostly outside the United States, continue to practice with unwritten, community-based ethics and seem to have no need for licenses, laws, and published codes. We value and respect different forms of midwifery practice without privileging one over another. We also acknowledge that some midwives in modern societies practice without documentation, certification, or licensure as "traditional midwives" and serve an important role, particularly in places where the practice of midwifery is not permitted by law. To say that they practice without ethical standards would be a mistake, for they are likely to share many ethical principles with licensed and certified practitioners. Nevertheless, midwives may face real and significant consequences for practicing without licensure or certification, particularly when complaints are lodged against them.

There has been a proliferation of midwifery organizations representing nurse–midwives and homebirth midwives, state associations, and international groups. What follows is a description of the major codes that have emerged from these groups, with a brief history of the guidelines that have been documented. We recognize that there are other codes of ethics and guidelines that may apply to some midwives (e.g., the American Nurses Association's Code of Ethics for Nurses). However, we focus our discussion on codes that were developed specifically for U.S. midwives, as well as the International Confederation of Midwives' code.

MIDWIVES ALLIANCE OF NORTH AMERICA STATEMENT OF VALUES AND ETHICS

The Midwives Alliance of North America (MANA) was founded in 1982 to set education and safety guidelines, facilitate communication, and establish a visible professional organization for all midwives, partly in response to the fact that many midwives were not eligible for membership in the American College of Nurse-Midwives (ACNM). A more complete history of MANA's birth can be found on the organization's Web site (MANA, 2005a).

MANA has published two documents related to ethical practice, neither of which is called an ethical code. Whereas the Statement of Values and Ethics (1997) (Appendix A) explicitly explores ethics and values related to midwifery, the Standards and Qualifications for the Art and Practice of Midwifery (2005b)

(Appendix B) give practical guidelines. According to Anne Frye (personal communication, July 15, 2009), former chair of the MANA Ethics Committee,

> the development of the MANA Statement of Values and Ethics was originally undertaken in the late 1980s to allow us to participate in the process of formulating a statement for the International Confederation of Midwives. Its creation involved broad member support and feedback. The revised version presented here was adopted in 1997. It was reviewed for this text, with minor typographical and grammatical changes incorporated.

Perhaps the most distinguishing feature of MANA's Statement of Values and Ethics is its acknowledgement of the limitations inherent in any code of ethics. MANA's statement opens with a brief introduction that is followed by six broad value areas: "Woman as an Individual with Unique Value and Worth," "Mother and Baby as a Whole," "The Nature of Birth," "The Art of Midwifery," "Woman as Mother," and "The Nature of Relationship." Each of these broad areas contains specific values (e.g., under "The Nature of Relationship": "We value honesty in relationships"). All together, the document contains 39 value statements. Note that the value statements do not directly state that midwives should or should not take any specific course of action. Although one might infer from the value of honesty that midwives should tell the truth, there are other value statements that do not have a clear behavioral corollary (e.g., "We value the essential mystery of birth").

Following the value statements, the MANA document contains some intriguing commentary on ethical codes, arguing that decision making is not facilitated by traditional codes, but rather is impaired by them. The authors of the document also implicate "the oppressive nature of the medical, legal or cultural framework in which we live" (p. 5).

MANA rejects rigid codes of ethics on several grounds, the first being that the rules and the skills needed to follow the codes are redundant. For example, MANA's statement suggests that the application of ethical codes requires capacities such as moral integrity and the ability to make judgments with adequate information, but that codes are rendered "superfluous" in the presence of these conditions. MANA also rejects ethical codes because they are deemed less reliable than practitioners. The statement takes the position that the practitioner's moral integrity is far more reliable than "a list of rules which must be followed" because "there cannot possibly be one right answer for all situations" (p. 5). In this respect, the MANA statement is consistent with the "context-sensitive approach" that we described in Chapter 1, recognizing that the realities of daily practice are incompatible with Western ethics' demand for objectivity and impartiality (Lützén, 1997, p. 218). Shortcomings of a purely contextual approach to ethics include ethical relativity, whereby no ethical or moral principle or theory is considered valid except as defined by culture or circumstance.

MANA's Statement of Values and Ethics does not merely reject conventional ethics, leaving midwives without guidance or direction. Rather, as an alternative to a code of ethics, MANA provides the value statements mentioned previously, along with a value-guided, process-oriented approach to ethical decision making. The document states that "ethics (how we act) proceed directly from a foundation of values" (p. 1). This value-guided approach to ethical behavior is summarized as follows (p. 6):

- Carefully defining our values
- Weighing the values in consideration with those of the community of midwives, families, and culture in which we find ourselves
- Acting in accord with our values to the best of our ability as the situation demands
- Engaging in ongoing self-examination and evaluation

The emphasis on values is noteworthy, particularly given the context in which you are likely reading this: as a student of ethics in midwifery. According to the MANA statement, the process of developing moral integrity and values cannot be taught, but rather must be acquired through personal growth. Ultimately, MANA turns responsibility for ethics over to midwives and pregnant women, "individual moral agents unique unto themselves . . . to follow and make known the dictates of our own consciences" (p. 6). Herein lies a paradox: MANA eschews rigid ethical guidelines in its Statement of Values and Ethics, yet establishes standards of practice in its Standards and Qualifications for the Art and Practice of Midwifery (2005b) that encompass ethical behavior that is commonly included in ethical codes.

Although the Standards and Qualifications document does not, on the surface, appear to serve the function of an ethical code, the guidelines contained therein resemble the elements of professional ethical codes. Moreover, MANA's Standards and Qualifications address informed choice, scope of practice, continuing education, and peer review, and they set clear behavioral expectations (e.g., "midwives will update their knowledge and skills on a regular basis" [n.p.]). In this regard, MANA's Statement of Values and Ethics should be conceptualized as a companion document to the Standards and Qualifications of the Art and Practice of Midwifery.

AMERICAN COLLEGE OF NURSE-MIDWIVES CODE OF ETHICS

With roots dating to 1929, the American College of Nurse-Midwives (ACNM) claims to be the oldest organization dedicated to women's health care in the

United States (ACNM, 2005). ACNM, which was incorporated in 1955, grew out of other organizations that failed to adequately represent the unique interests of midwifery. A detailed history can be found on the ACNM's Web site (ACNM, 2005).

The ACNM publishes two versions of its code of ethics, both of which were reviewed and endorsed by the ACNM Ethics Committee in 2008. The shorter version is a one-page document that lists 11 ethical standards that are divided into three sections: professional relationships, professional practice, and responsibilities to the profession of midwifery. The longer version, *The American College of Nurse-Midwives Code of Ethics with Explanatory Statements* (Appendix C), maintains the same 11 standards but also offers considerable commentary (this version is 18 pages long).

The long version contains an introduction that places the document in context. The opening paragraphs note that the ACNM code contains "moral obligations" that "reflect universal ethical principles that are traditionally associated with the health-care professions but have been written to emphasize midwifery values and standards" (ACNM, 2008, p. 1). Recall that in Chapter 1, we addressed some of these broad ethical principles and identified professional differentiation as one benefit of developing ethical codes. ACNM makes explicit the relationship between existing healthcare principles and also maintains that midwifery is unique.

The long version of ACNM's code makes clear the various purposes of the document. The code guides midwifery practice, provides direction to students of midwifery regarding moral obligations, facilitates peer review and consultation, and educates others (e.g., the public) about the profession's ethical guidelines. Collectively, these purposes help midwifery maintain professional integrity (ACNM, 2008).

A word of caution precedes the core content of ACNM's code: the moral obligations may be in conflict with one another and are not absolute. When ethical dilemmas arise, midwives are encouraged to consider the impact of decisions on all potentially affected parties and to consider the context of the particular situation (ACNM, 2008). However, note that unlike MANA's Statement of Values and Ethics, the ACNM Code of Ethics makes clear statements regarding not only values but also behaviors.

The first two obligations in the ACNM's code fall under the category of professional relationships. Midwives "respect basic human rights and the dignity of all persons" and "respect their own self worth, dignity, and professional integrity" (pp. 3–4). If you were reading the short version of the Code of Ethics, you would find no further explanation or guidance regarding these obligations. Fortunately, the long version provides some elaboration that greatly enhances the quality of the document.

The ACNM Code of Ethics states that these first two moral obligations concerning professional relationships serve as a foundation for the remaining nine moral obligations listed. The explanatory statement goes on to note that respect for human rights and dignity relates directly to established notions of valuing autonomy and justice (e.g., the United Nations Declaration of Human Rights, 1948), but highlights the fact that these rights historically have not been equally afforded to females. As a matter of beneficence and justice, midwives work to prevent violations of women's rights at the micro level (individuals served) and macro level (through policy and legal reforms). They respect others who have different values and opinions, even if they do not agree with those viewpoints. The foundation of the relationship is built on "trust, integrity, truth-telling, compassion, caring, and respect" (p. 4). Relationships with clients, students, other providers, policy makers, administrators, and anyone else served by a midwife fall under this obligation of respect.

Respecting the dignity of others, the first ACNM ethical obligation, requires little explanation or elaboration and overlaps considerably with established ethical standards. However, the second obligation regarding self-worth is not so straightforward. The explanatory statement helps place this item in context for application in real-world practice. If one were to look only at the short version of the ACNM code, the full meaning of "self worth, dignity, and professional integrity" would not be apparent. Although this standard is ostensibly about midwives, the explanatory document reveals a subtler perspective of self (midwife) and others. "Respect of self worth and dignity" means that midwives must "respect their own values and competences in interaction with others and seek alternative solutions to prevent compromise of important professional principles, values and goals" (p. 4). Essentially, this standard addresses the need for the midwife to balance her own autonomy with the rights and needs of others. For example, midwives sometimes experience conflict in maintaining integrity with respect to their professional standards while simultaneously meeting their clients' needs for autonomy and self-direction.

The second set of obligations (3 through 8) focuses on serving women and their families and the public good. The third moral obligation states that midwives "develop a partnership with the woman in which each shares relevant information that leads to informed decision-making, consent to an evolving plan of care, and acceptance of responsibility for the outcome of their choices" (p. 6). In this statement, the ACNM code addresses informed consent or informed choice, discussed extensively in Chapter 4 of this text. At the outset of services, the midwife ensures that the client understands the risks and benefits of midwifery care before voluntarily consenting to accept care from a midwife. Moreover, this part of the code emphasizes shared responsibility, which is to say that both the midwife and the client are invested in and responsible for the quality of care. Information sharing from all parties is recognized as a critical component of shared responsibility.

The fourth moral obligation is for midwives to "act without discrimination based on factors such as age, gender, race, ethnicity, religion, lifestyle, sexual orientation, socioeconomic status, disability, or nature of the health problem" (p. 8). Midwives maintain adherence to principles of justice by treating all clients fairly and equally, and also advocating for their clients in the face of institutional discriminatory practices (e.g., a hospital's refusal to treat a lesbian partner as a spouse). Midwives are encouraged to be aware of their own biases and take steps to maintain equality in the care they provide.

Privacy and confidentiality are addressed by statements 5 and 6 of the ACNM Code of Ethics and are discussed in detail in Chapter 3 of this text. The code recognizes that situational and contextual factors can present challenges to maintaining privacy and confidentiality. For example, when an interpreter is used for a client who does not speak the same language as her care providers, midwives must ensure that the interpreter respects the client's confidentiality. In some hospital settings, women may feel that insufficient measures have been taken to provide privacy, and midwives advocate for increased protections.

Maintaining competence in midwifery knowledge and skills falls under the broad ethical principle of responsible caring and is the seventh obligation in ACNM's code. Midwives are expected to continually assess their own competency and take steps to increase and update their knowledge and skills as the art and science of midwifery evolve. Knowing the limits of one's competency is also critical, because midwives should not engage in practices that are outside their skill set. When a midwife is presented with care scenarios that test the limits of her competency, she is advised to seek consultation and supervision from another clinician or refer the client to a provider who has the necessary skills to provide appropriate care.

In the interest of protecting clients from harm, midwives have an obligation to take "appropriate action" to protect others from "harmful, unethical, and incompetent practices" (p. 12). Taking moral obligations beyond a "do no harm" approach, this eighth statement in ACNM's code instructs midwives to report harmful practices to the appropriate authorities in the interest of protecting clients, their families, and colleagues. Harm is described as "adverse physical, emotional, psychological, social or economic effects of practices or behaviors" (p. 12). Such harms can occur not only through clinical care but also through business practices, education, and research.

The final section of the ACNM Code of Ethics contains three statements that address the profession and mission of midwifery, with obligations to both the profession and the public. The first statement notes that midwives are members of a professional community who "promote, advocate for, and strive to protect the rights, health, and well-being of women, families and communities" (p. 14). Here, the responsibilities to clients and families are emphasized less than the responsibilities to work at policy and societal levels. In a similar vein, the second statement in this section addresses just distribution of healthcare resources: midwives "promote just distribution of resources and equity in access to quality health services" (p. 16). Noting that health care is a human right, ACNM takes a strong position that midwives should work to ensure that everyone has equal access to health care.

The final statement listed in the ACNM Code of Ethics concerns the promotion and support of "the education of midwifery students and peers, standards of practice, research and policies that enhance the health of women, families and communities" (p. 16). Here, ACNM defines health very broadly to encompass mental health and social well-being. Promoting research and education can take many forms, including the use of research-based practices and the mentoring of midwifery students. The emphasis of this standard is clearly on the midwife's responsibilities for health promotion at the profession level rather than the individual level.

INTERNATIONAL CODE OF ETHICS FOR MIDWIVES

The International Confederation of Midwives (ICM) represents over 90 midwifery organizations from 80 countries. Founded in 1919 by European midwives, the ICM has held meetings every three years for decades. Based in the Netherlands, ICM publishes the journal *International Midwifery*. A more detailed history can be found on ICM's Web site (ICM, 2008).

The ICM adopted a code of ethics in 1993 that encompasses midwifery relationships, practice, professional behavior, and the advancement of midwifery knowledge and practice. The first document was drafted over a series of workshops, beginning in 1987. The final document was passed by full consensus in the ICM Executive Committee before being adopted by the ICM Council. The code has been revised, most recently in 2003, and reflects the aims and values of ICM in terms of improving maternity and family care, upholding equity and justice in health care, and fostering mutual relationships of respect, trust, and dignity. Composed of 21 statements descriptive of midwifery values and ethical guidelines, ICM's International Code of Ethics for Midwives (ICM, 2003) (Appendix D) is intended to guide education, practice, and research in the field of midwifery.

Under the heading of "Midwifery Relationships," the ICM code describes how midwives relate to their clients, work in communities, advocate for fair healthcare policies, interact with other midwives, collaborate with other healthcare professionals, and protect themselves. Client relationships are outlined in areas of informed choice and active participation in care. The language is descriptive, such as "midwives respect a woman's informed right of choice and promote the woman's acceptance of responsibility for the outcome of her choices" (ICM, 2003, p. 1). In the context of community work, the ICM code describes midwives as being collaborative healthcare activists in the areas of policies and allocation of resources, while empowering women to become advocates for themselves and their families in health care. ICM's code also explains the interdependence of midwives and their related responsibilities to resolve differences and provide support for one another. This statement is highly salient to marginalized midwives, who are often defined by the political context in which they practice. Similarly, midwives are said to maintain positive professional relationships for the interest of midwifery. The code further defines professional conduct: "Midwives work with other health professionals, consulting and referring as necessary when the woman's need for care exceeds the competencies of the midwife" (p. 1). This statement recognizes the need for midwives to work within a "scope of practice" that is limited by licensure, education, experience, and knowledge.

The second section of the International Code of Ethics for Midwives focuses on the practice of midwifery. Under this heading, midwifery behavior is described as respectful of diversity, protective of childbearing women, responsible for ensuring safe birthing practices, and holistic. Midwifery practice is an essential resource for the birthing community, and as such, the ICM code places the midwife in a central position to affect cultural change regarding childbearing. Midwives are charged with care of the woman beyond her physical being, responding to her emotional and spiritual needs as well. "Midwives act as effective role models in health promotion for women throughout their life cycle, for families and for other health professionals" (p. 2). Finally, midwives are charged with the task of personal, intellectual, and professional development.

The International Code of Ethics for Midwives deals with professional responsibilities by addressing confidentiality and responsibility for the outcomes of provided care. Affirmation of the practitioner's right to moral opposition to unnamed practices is balanced with a woman's right to healthcare services. Further, midwives are called to work toward eliminating human rights violations. For a second time in the code, midwives are called to develop and implement healthcare policies to serve women and families.

Finally, under the heading "Advancement of Midwifery Knowledge and Practice," ICM's code grounds midwifery knowledge in actively "protect[ing] the rights of women as persons" (p. 2). To advance midwifery, midwives are involved in formal and continuing education for midwifery students and midwives, as well as peer review and research.

NATIONAL ASSOCIATION OF CERTIFIED PROFESSIONAL MIDWIVES

The National Association of Certified Professional Midwives (NACPM) was formed in 2000 to support the professional development of Certified Professional Midwives (CPMs). In 2002, NACPM elected its first board of directors and formed committees to develop standards of practice, incorporating input from its membership. The Essential Documents, which function in part as a code of ethics and set of practice standards, were adopted in 2004.

Following a brief introduction, the NACPM Essential Documents (Appendix E) are divided into the following sections: "Philosophy and Principles of Practice," "Scope of Practice," "Standards of Practice for NACPM Members," and "Endorsement of Supportive Statements." The purpose of the documents is to identify core values, definitions of practice, ethical guidelines, and philosophical orientation. Although NACPM does not refer to the Essential Documents as a code of ethics, we treat it as such in this text.

The "Philosophy and Principles of Practice" is basically an affirmation and reiteration of the MMOC (e.g., women-centered care, normalcy of birth, the oneness of mother and child, birth as a spiritual event). Additionally, it includes aspects of clinical judgment, evidence-based care, and limitations of midwifery practice. The philosophy section ends with a recognition that midwives serve women through a collaboration with or referral to other care providers, which sometimes includes medical practitioners.

The next section, "Scope of Practice," is only one paragraph. However, that paragraph covers a wide range of topics. It defines the scope of practice and expertise of NACPM members, noting that they "offer expert care, education, counseling and support to women and their families throughout the caregiving partnership, including pregnancy, birth and the postpartum period" (NACPM, 2004, p. 2). Informed consent is highlighted as an essential component of client education and counseling (for more on informed consent, see Chapter 4). The role of midwives in seeking appropriate consultation and in providing referral and emergency care is explained.

The bulk of the document is in the "Standards of Practice" section, consisting of six standards with explanatory statements. Overall, the standards reflect ethical considerations, MMOC values, and guidelines for competency and professional development. Although these are presented as standards, they are behavioral and instructive in nature. They reflect the values of NACPM and simultaneously provide specific practice guidelines.

The first standard locates the responsibility of care within the midwife-client partnership, with respect for the woman's autonomy in making decisions and taking responsibility for her own health care. The midwife's role as educator, care provider, and counselor is emphasized, as well as her duty to provide informed consent and uphold professional boundaries. Respect for the woman's dignity is expressed through individualized care without imposition of values. This demonstrates NACPM's value of diversity.

Standard 2 focuses on the nature of midwifery practice. It includes continuity of care, evidence-based practices, competency in emergencies, appropriate referrals, and collaborations. Further, this section includes the midwife's responsibility for self-care. In sum, the section upholds the caring quality of midwifery and outlines related professional responsibilities.

The third standard includes ethical responsibilities related to informed consent, scope of practice, and transfer of care. It instructs the midwife to maintain clear communication with clients in order to uphold informed choice. It provides guidelines for addressing conflicts in the clinical relationship and clear indications for termination of care. Upholding safety is an underpinning value in this section.

Standard 4 instructs the midwife in the closure of the clinical relationship. Midwives provide care to women through the final postnatal appointment unless the woman chooses to terminate care sooner. Midwives ensure that women have the capacity to care for themselves and their infant prior to discharge. Further, midwives provide an opportunity for each woman to review her birth experience. The standard directs midwives to provide community resources to clients at the end of care.

Privacy is the main concern addressed in the fifth standard of the NACPM's Essential Documents. Directives are provided to ensure proper documentation, including the use of individualized assessments as a guide to ongoing care. Women should have open access to their own personal health records and exercise control over other's access to those records. NACPM upholds confidentiality as a standard for midwifery care.

The final standard relates to the midwife's professional development, skills, and competency, stating that "the midwife continuously evaluates and improves her knowledge, skills and practice in her endeavor to provide the best possible care" (p. 4). NACPM members are expected to incorporate client feedback, practice statistics, continuing education, peer review, and research findings into an overall plan of growth and improvement. Additionally, this standard expects members to influence social policies related to the health of mothers and babies.

Following these six practice standards, NACPM's Essential Documents contains a brief endorsement of the MMOC, the Mother Friendly Childbirth Initiative (Coalition for Improving Maternity Services, 1996), and the Rights of Childbearing Women (Childbirth Connection, 2004). NACPM provides no commentary regarding these endorsements, but refers readers to Web sites that contain the full text of each statement.

ANALYSIS OF THE MIDWIFERY CODES

Numerous similarities among the aforementioned codes bind them together as reflections of deeply held values espoused by modern practicing midwives regardless of training, professional affiliations, and location of practice. This validates the values that are arguably inherent to the practice of midwifery, including dignity for persons, respect for women's autonomy, working in partnership with the women we serve, protecting self-worth and informed choice, furthering midwifery knowledge, and providing equity in care. These tenets are echoed by ACNM, MANA, ICM, and NACPM and convey midwives' deep commitment to providing quality services grounded in caring for women and their families.

In contrasting the codes, the absence of specific ethical considerations is striking. ICM's failure to attend to the issue of midwifery skills, and the absence of any mention of privacy or confidentiality in MANA's statement are noteworthy. Refer to Table 2-1 for further analysis of code content across various ethical considerations. Only ICM directly addresses the challenging ethical dilemma of potentially harmful cultural practices, where respect for cultural diversity is tried: "Midwives provide care for women and childbearing families with respect for cultural diversity while also working to eliminate harmful practices within those same cultures," clearly showing the insights of an international organization (ICM, 2003, p. 2).

The ACNM Code of Ethics (2008) and NACPM's Essential Documents (2004) go furthest in terms of descriptive actions for practice. For example, the ACNM code provides the following directive: "Protect women, their families, and colleagues from harmful, unethical, incompetent practices by taking appropriate action that may include reporting as mandated by law" (ACNM, 2008, p.12). The long version of the ACNM code provides guidelines that are essential to the practitioner. In the introduction, moral conflicts are addressed with specified areas of consideration, including contextual factors, the goal of consensus among involved parties prior to action, and ethical compromise. Abstract words contained in the code are defined in the long version. For example, "respect" is "when people are able to determine the courses of action they will take and accept accountability for the outcome of these choices . . . Respect does not imply automatic agreement with another's decisions or actions, nor does it relieve midwives of the obligation to protect others and themselves when choices may cause harm" (ACNM, 2008, p. 3). The long version does much to enhance the practical application of the Code of Ethics of the American College of Nurse-Midwives.

NACPM's Essential Documents (2004) also provides specific guidelines. For example, the midwife "does not impose her value system on the woman" (p. 2). Rather than making a general statement about values and respect, this docu-

Table 2-1   A Comparison of the Codes or Value Statements of ICM, MANA, ACNM, and NACPM

Statement or Value	ICM	MANA	ACNM	NACPM
Promotes woman's acceptance of responsibility for outcomes of her choices	•		•	•
Clearly identifies fees for services				•
Equity in access to health care for all	•		•	
Justice for all	•		•	
Informed consent	•	•	•	•
Privacy	•		•	•
Confidentiality	•		•	•
Professional competency	•	•	•	•
Professional relationships	•	•	•	
Fidelity and responsibility			•	•
Integrity		•	•	
Justice			•	
Conflicts of interest			•	•
Cooperation with other professionals	•		•	•
Advertising and other public statements			•	
Recognizes and attempts to compensate for language barriers			•	•
Proper documentation			•	•
Uses practice statistics and feedback from women to improve practice of midwifery				•
Continued education and training		•	•	•

(continues)

Table 2-1   A Comparison of the Codes or Value Statements of ICM, MANA, ACNM, and NACPM *(continued)*

Statement or Value	ICM	MANA	ACNM	NACPM
Shares research findings and incorporates them into practice as appropriate			•	•
Respect for autonomy (of client)	•	•	•	•
Continued self-assessment		•	•	•
Respects diversity	•	•	•	•
Responds to psychological, physical, emotional, and spiritual needs of women	•	•		•
Respects the importance of others in the woman's life	•	•	•	•
Awareness of policies and laws			•	•
Promotes, advocates, and strives to protect rights of women, families, and community	•	•	•	•
Pursues fairness, justness, and equity	•		•	
Acts in accord with values to best of ability	•	•	•	
Respects own self-worth	•	•	•	•
Self-care				•
Values the oneness of the pregnant mother and unborn child		•		•
Values the birth experience as a rite of passage		•		•
Values the integrity of natural birth		•		•
Values the breastfeeding relationship		•		
Values the mystery of birth		•		•
Facilitates informed decision making	•		•	•
Values the empowerment of women in all aspects of life		•	•	

ment takes the additional step of setting a limit on the midwife's behavior. Further, the document states that the midwife "maintains her own health and well-being to optimize her ability to provide care" (p. 3). This acknowledges the necessity of the caregiver's commitment to personal care and its relationship to caring for others with specific guidelines. There are very specific behavioral components to documentation and privacy as well. For example, "the NACPM member . . . does not share the woman's medical and midwifery records without her permission except as medically required" (p. 4).

The ACNM code reflects a deep understanding of the need for an ethical code in midwifery. Its content contrasts with that of the MANA and ICM codes in meaningful ways that may reflect a greater emphasis on the identity of the midwife as a professional healthcare provider. It does not concur with ICM's position in preserving a woman's access to healthcare services when an individual midwife is morally opposed to participating in an activity or practice. Rather, the midwife is discouraged from sacrificing her own moral integrity, and referral is recommended. This difference demonstrates the contrast between these two organizations, one of which is international.

The ICM code (2003) clearly mirrors the historical context in which it was created. During the late 1980s and early 1990s, the values of cultural diversity and political correctness became the standards by which language was judged. International midwives gathered during this time to analyze existing ethical codes as a first step. A great effort was taken by the composers of the code to maintain cultural sensitivity. Further effort was made to uphold global or universal morality, while avoiding legal references. These goals allowed the emergence of a body of ethical values that reflects an enlightened, educated, and pluralistic moral system espoused by international midwives. The voices of the midwives and their place and time are effective in identifying core midwifery values, even as the code falls short in prescribing ethical conduct.

By avoiding concrete ethical guidance, the ICM document lacks utility in real-world practice. The language of the document is more akin to a mission statement than a practical ethical code. The code's content reflects the MMOC's concern with women's personal responsibility and informed choice, but does little to direct the practicing midwife in applying these principles. Similarly, MANA's statement offers limited guidance for application in a real-world practice.

A feminist deconstruction of ethics, MANA's Statement of Values and Ethics eloquently defies the status quo for applied ethics that is deduced by abstract principles largely derived from male-dominated fields and ivory-tower academicians. In so doing, MANA mirrors late 20th-century feminist philosophies, such as Carol Gilligan's popularized study of women's moral thinking, *In a Different Voice* (1993), and Mary Field Belenky and colleagues' *Women's Ways of Knowing* (1986), a supportive analysis of essential feministic views on gendered cognition and communication.

In deconstructing ethical codes, MANA has purposefully left little structure for ethical judgments and actions, providing midwives with enviable clinical freedom. Are midwives above ethics? Clearly, MANA trusts midwives to make good, ethical choices, much like the MMOC trusts women to do the same. This approach is not without drawbacks. Leaving midwives to make ethical decisions in context without practical guidelines may allow for too much flexibility and could potentially fail to protect the people we serve and the profession we hold so dear. Midwives should be held to the highest standard of ethics to reflect our commitment to childbearing women and their families and our dedication to feminist core values.

MANA's Statement of Values and Ethics (1997) has some of the strongest language in terms of quality of care and respect for autonomy of women and their choices. The MMOC is clearly reflected in each section of the document, with thoughtful inclusion of midwifery concepts reflecting the sanctity of birth, the oneness of mother and child, the art of midwifery and personal responsibility. Informed choice and women's abilities and rights as mothers are emphasized in multiple locations in the statement. The feminist orientation of this document is an asset to the essential body of literature in midwifery, yet as an ethical code, it does not provide sufficient guidance, referencing only a few polarized resources (e.g., *Gyn Ecology: The Metaethics of Radical Feminism, Lesbian Ethics: Toward New Value,* and *Going Out of Our Minds: The Metaphysics of Liberation*). These resources represent an ideological perspective sometimes referred to as radical feminist thought, an arguably appropriate reaction to dominant Western male paradigms. The MANA statement is currently in revision, and we anticipate improvements to the existing document. As stated earlier, MANA's Standards and Qualifications for the Art and Practice for Midwifery (2005) picks up ethical guidelines that MANA's Statement of Values and Ethics leaves out.

Taken together, the four codes covered in this chapter offer wide-ranging ethical guidance, from deeply held values consistent among all three midwifery associations to specific guidelines for maintaining confidentiality, informed consent, and ethical decision making. They are each valuable documents for their organizations. ACNM and NACPM offer the greatest resources to their members by providing practical guidelines. The ICM and MANA each developed codes that reflect their membership identity, yet which are less useful for midwifery practices. A midwife affiliated with any of these organizations should, at the least, be aware of the appropriate ethical code(s) and, at best, attend regular training in ethics and use ethical guidelines in daily practice, while supporting the development of ethics in the field.

Whereas other fields that interface intimately with the public, such as psychology, medicine, and social work, require their members to take ethical classes as part of their training and often require the attendance of regular ethics workshops (as determined by licensing and credentialing boards, typically), midwives are usually exempted from such regulation. This may be an oversight of the current milieu, where the battles for licensure and scope of practice take center stage and midwives struggle for professional validation in a healthcare system dominated by medical doctors, insurance companies, and hospital administrators.

It is our belief that strengthening our ethical codes and deepening our commitment to ethical training will protect the professional autonomy of midwives, assist midwives in promoting the profession, and increase respect for midwives among other healthcare professionals. Most important, a strong working knowledge of applied ethics will improve midwifery care for women and their families.

A number of possible avenues exist for reaching the goal of strengthening ethics in midwifery. The aforementioned codes may be strengthened. The individual midwife may voluntarily seek training in ethics and use her knowledge in her practice. Midwifery organizations may elect to hold regular training in ethics at conferences. Midwifery schools may take the lead by offering ethics courses and requiring completion of ethics training for graduation. Finally, regulatory bodies, such as the state midwifery boards, may add requirements for ethical training in order to be recertified or licensed. It is likely that each of these steps will be necessary to fully integrate applied ethics into the field of midwifery. See Chapter 11 for further suggestions regarding proactive ethics.

As a student, practitioner, or instructor in the field, it may be up to you to assist the growth of midwifery in this direction. The existing codes have set the foundation on which to build applied ethics. As stated earlier in this chapter, the codes convey midwives' deep commitment to providing quality services grounded in caring for women and their families. This commitment to caring is what is likely to drive the development of ethics in midwifery. Fortunately, it is a potentially unlimited resource.

REFERENCES

American College of Nurse-Midwives (ACNM). (2005). *About us*. Retrieved January 30, 2009, from http://www.acnm.org/about.cfm

American College of Nurse-Midwives (ACNM). (2008). *American College of Nurse-Midwives code of ethics with explanatory statements*. Silver Spring, MD: Author.

Belenky, M. F., Clinchy, B. M., Goldberg, N. R., & Tarule, J. M. (1986). *Women's ways of knowing: The development of self, voice, and mind*. New York: Basic Books.

Childbirth Connection. (2004). *The rights of childbearing women*. New York: Author.

Coalition for Improving Maternity Services (CIMS). (1996). *Mother friendly childbirth initiative*. Raleigh, NC: Author.

Gilligan, C. (1993). *In a different voice*. Cambridge, MA: Harvard University Press.

International Confederation of Midwives (ICM). (2003). *ICM international code of ethics for midwives*. Retrieved January 30, 2009, from http://www.internationalmidwives.org/Documentation/Coredocuments/tabid/322/Default.aspx

International Confederation of Midwives (ICM). (2008). *A short history of the ICM*. Retrieved January 30, 2009, from http://www.internationalmidwives.org/AboutICM/History/tabid/338/Default.aspx

Lopez Lysne, R. (2006). The very oldest profession. *Midwifery Today, 78*, 48–49.

Lützén, K. (1997). Nursing ethics into the next millennium: A context-sensitive approach for nursing ethics. *Nursing Ethics, 4*(3), 218–226.

Midwives Alliance of North America (MANA). (1997). *Statement of values and ethics*. Washington, DC: Author.

Midwives Alliance of North America (MANA). (2005a). *MANA news supplement*. Retrieved January 30, 2009, from http://mana.org/history.html

Midwives Alliance of North America (MANA). (2005b). *Standards and qualifications for the art and practice of midwifery*. Washington, DC: Author.

National Association of Certified Professional Midwives (NACPM). (2004). *Essential documents*. Retrieved August 1, 2009, from http://www.nacpm.org/Resources/nacpm-standards.pdf

Rothman, B. K. (1979). *Two models in maternity care: Defining and negotiating reality*. New York: New York University Press.

United Nations (UN). (1948). *The Universal Declaration of Human Rights*. Retrieved December 8, 2008, from http://www.un.org/Overview/rights.html

CHAPTER 3

Privacy and Confidentiality

Midwives have both ethical and legal responsibilities regarding privacy and confidentiality (Tschudin, 2003). Although midwives have always been sensitive to issues regarding personal health information, changes in technology, culture, and law have presented new challenges and heightened client and practitioner awareness of these issues (Aiken, 2009; Ives Erickson & Millar, 2005). Unfortunately, many changes in technology have outpaced changes to laws and policies. This chapter provides an overview of privacy and confidentiality, followed by practical guidelines for daily practice and case examples.

FOUNDATIONS OF PRIVACY

Consistent with broad ethical principles concerning respect and responsible caring, midwives recognize clients' privacy rights. As mentioned earlier, midwives respect the dignity of all people and apply this standard to their professional work. One extension of this principle is respect for the privacy of others. Privacy is considered a basic human right, and as such has been enumerated in the United Nations' Universal Declaration of Human Rights (1948): "No one shall be subjected to arbitrary interference with his [sic] privacy, family, home or correspondence, nor to attacks upon his [sic] honour and reputation." As with many key concepts in this book, privacy has both legal and ethical foundations.

The legal roots of privacy in the United States can be traced back to the Declaration of Independence (e.g., the right to "life, liberty, and the pursuit of happiness") as well as the United States Constitution (e.g., the Fourth Amendment's guarantee that "the right of the people to be secure in their persons, houses, papers and effects, against unreasonable searches and seizures, shall not be violated"). Curiously, the word *privacy* does not appear in the Constitution. Nevertheless, the Supreme Court has maintained that a right to privacy can be inferred from other enumerated rights.

The case of *Griswold v. Connecticut* (1965), which reached the U.S. Supreme Court, questioned the constitutionality of a law that prohibited the distribution of contraception, even to married couples. In the Court's opinion, Justice

Douglas wrote that case law suggests "that specific guarantees in the Bill of Rights have penumbras, formed by emanations from those guarantees that help give them life and substance." In other words, the right to privacy, although not explicitly stated, has been inferred from other enumerated rights. According to Douglas, privacy could be derived from, among other rights, the First Amendment's freedom of assembly, the Third Amendment's protection against soldiers quartering in our homes during peacetime, and the Fourth Amendment's protection from unreasonable searches and seizures.

This right to privacy, even if it is not mentioned directly by name in the Constitution, is widely respected and cherished. All 50 states recognize a right to privacy, providing even further legal support. We must bear in mind that the legal right to privacy is not an absolute right. Even though we have protections from unreasonable searches and seizures, the government may have legitimate reasons to search our homes (e.g., with a warrant for a criminal investigation). The fact that limitations on privacy rights exist suggests that the need for privacy must be balanced with other competing needs, such as public safety and welfare. For example, the Health Insurance Portability and Accountability Act of 1996 (HIPAA) notes that although there are many protections to keep health records private, care providers must report health information to prevent the transmission of communicable diseases (U.S. Department of Health and Human Services, n.d.), and the Privacy Act of 1974 contains exceptions for law enforcement. Similarly, healthcare providers must reveal private health information to the authorities if they suspect abuse (e.g., upon the discovery of bruises on a child following a routine physical examination).

Most likely, the development of legal protection for privacy originated in the moral principles associated with privacy, such as respect for the dignity and autonomy of others. As mentioned in Chapter 1, the principle of nonmaleficence directs us to avoid causing harm to others. There are a number of midwifery scenarios in which the failure to respect a client's privacy could result in harm. For example, a client may disclose to a midwife in the course of her medical history that she has had an abortion, but does not want her husband to know about it. Should the midwife disregard the client's right to control this information, she runs the risk of harming the marital relationship and the midwife-client relationship.

Respecting the privacy of clients also speaks to the general values of the Midwives Model of Care (MMOC) (Rothman, 1979), which empowers clients by placing them in control of their pregnancy and birth. Control over personal health information is an important extension of this notion of empowerment. To fulfill this obligation well, midwives must take the time needed to explain to clients why personal information is collected and how it will be stored, shared, and maintained. The midwife must explain to the client her rights, as well as any limitations of those rights (a topic we will address more thoroughly later in this chapter in the context of confidentiality).

PRIVACY VERSUS CONFIDENTIALITY

Privacy and *confidentiality* are related terms that have similar, yet distinct, meanings (Ives Erickson & Millar, 2005). Privacy refers to the client's right to control her own information. When a client shares private information, the midwife has an obligation to regard the information as confidential and to treat it as such by limiting disclosure to others under specific circumstances. Therefore, privacy is a client's right, and confidentiality is a midwife's obligation. Just as privacy is circumscribed by both ethical and legal standards, so too the duty to maintain confidentiality comes from more than one source.

CONFIDENTIALITY

All of the major organizations in midwifery have addressed confidentiality and privacy in their professional documents. The *Code of Ethics with Explanatory Statements* of the American College of Nurse-Midwives (ACNM) states that "Midwives in all aspects of their professional practice will maintain confidentiality except where disclosure is mandated by law" (ACNM, 2004, p. 10; see Appendix C). The code of the International Confederation of Midwives (ICM) includes guidelines for confidentiality as well: "Midwives hold in confidence client information in order to protect the right to privacy and use judgment in sharing this information" (ICM, 2003, p. 2; see Appendix D). In its Essential Documents, the National Association of Certified Professional Midwives (NACPM) states that "the NACPM member . . . does not share the woman's medical and midwifery records without her permission, except as legally required" (NACPM, 2004, p. 4; see Appendix E). Confidentiality is also addressed in the Midwives Alliance of North America's (MANA) Standards and Qualifications for the Art and Practice of Midwifery (MANA, 2005; see Appendix B). What follows is a more general discussion of salient issues related to the protections of personal information in midwifery.

Midwives have an ethical and legal responsibility to treat private and personal client information with great care and respect. Client information may be verbal or written (e.g., medical records). Midwives also collect client data through physical examinations and lab reports, which must also be treated as confidential. Only under limited circumstances involving proper care management and documentation should a midwife share client information. For example, with her client's consent, a midwife could share lab results with a perinatologist in the interest of facilitating the client's care. Both federal and state laws mandate that healthcare providers ensure the confidentiality of client information. Therefore, an inappropriate breach of confidentiality could result in both an ethical violation as well as legal action. In keeping with the focus of this book, we emphasize the ethical issues regarding confidentiality.

Clients come to midwives with expectations and assumptions about their personal health information. When a client exercises her privacy rights by choosing to share sensitive data with her midwife, she trusts that the midwife will treat the data with great care. A clear discussion of confidentiality must take place before services are initiated and before the client discloses personal information. The midwife has two primary obligations to the client at this point in care: to inform the client that her information will not be shared without the client's consent and to communicate the limitations of confidentiality to the client.

Even information shared by a client that is unrelated to her care is expected to be held in confidence (Aiken, 2009). A midwife must balance her obligation to her client with other legitimate needs, however. For example, when a client shares that her abusive husband has injured their child, the midwife has a duty to report the abuse to protective services. Because clients often assume that their disclosures will remain confidential under all circumstances, it behooves the midwife to make such limits to confidentiality known from the start.

Earlier we noted in our discussion of privacy that clients have the right to control their information. One way that they can exercise this right is by giving a midwife permission to share personal information with others. For example, a postpartum mother who is having trouble breastfeeding may be referred to a lactation consultant. With the mother's written consent, the midwife may share client data with the lactation consultant. In such situations, midwives and clients should discuss how much information should be shared with a third party and make such agreements explicit. What follows is a discussion of privacy and confidentiality as applied to the real-world practice of midwifery.

PRIVACY AND CONFIDENTIALITY IN PRACTICE

In professional health care, maintaining confidentiality is central to the protection of the public. Health professionals maintain confidentiality by protecting client records, communications with clients and their family members, and other personal information in a variety of settings. When a woman seeks the care of a midwife, she expects this level of professionalism, which is due to her both ethically and legally. To fulfill our role for the women we serve, midwives must develop and utilize a policy to maintain privacy and confidentiality.

The consequences of confidentiality and privacy breaches cannot be underestimated. When personal health information is not protected, providers could jeopardize clients' insurability, employment, and relationships (Aiken, 2009). Midwives and other healthcare providers may become habituated to sensitive health information as a result of frequent exposure, but must be mindful of the fact that each individual client has the right to privacy and that every provider has a responsibility to maintain information and records in such a way that protects her or his clients.

Client Records

Proper storage and accessibility of client records is essential in maintaining confidentiality in the midwife-client relationship. Records should be stored behind locked doors or in a locked cabinet, and electronic records must be password protected. Access to patient records within a practice or among hospital professionals must be limited to professionals on a "need to know" basis (Aiken, 2009). Jones (2000) states that by virtue of giving information to a care provider with the knowledge that the information has been recorded, a client essentially gives "implied consent" that the information can be shared with other providers on a need-to-know basis. We disagree and believe that midwives should seek the informed consent of their clients before releasing information to other care providers whenever possible (see Chapter 4 on informed consent). We recognize that in many practice settings, Jones's notion of implied consent prevails. Nevertheless, unless situational factors dictate otherwise, limited access to records is most consistent with ethical standards.

Tschudin (2003) notes that exceptions to rules about confidentiality can be sources of confusion and may indeed result in harm. She illustrates the challenges to a practitioner when there are exceptions to the rules of confidentiality with an example from the Nursing and Midwifery Council's (2002) code (Appendix F). This code suggests that in some cases not all of the information that a client gives to a nurse or midwife is necessarily protected. Exceptions to confidentiality may reflect local confidentiality policies. When midwives have doubts about confidentiality issues, they should review existing codes and local standards and consult with trusted colleagues.

Maintaining and controlling the accessibility of client records requires a privacy policy that is communicated to clients. The privacy policy must reflect ethical codes and local guidelines, as well as policies and restrictions for access to client records, including HIPAA (1996), where applicable. Clients should be made aware that exceptions to HIPAA rules require healthcare providers to give medical records to the government without prior patient authorization for "national security" reasons (Kumekawa, 2005). A practice's privacy policy should disclose how clients can access their files and how health information is shared. In communicating your privacy policy to a client, you are acknowledging her inherent right to privacy, your respect for her integrity, and her right to access her private health records.

HIPPA requires healthcare providers to permit individuals to access their personal healthcare records. Some midwives offer clients access to their files at each prenatal visit by inviting women to chart their own weight. In many settings, this level of accessibility would be impractical or might result in the accidental disclosure of private information. Yet this practice reflects the MMOC in that it places the woman at the center of her care; she becomes a collaborative member of her healthcare team. Her records are accessible to her because they belong to her. The midwife maintains the chart as a way to organize and record a woman's care on her behalf. This is a major departure from a typical medical-model policy for patient files, which are kept in the hands of the nurses or the office staff in a doctor's office and where a woman must often wait at least a month if she wants a copy of her records. Midwives can do much to improve clients' access to records to further emphasize the MMOC and woman-centered maternity care.

Disclosures

The midwife maintains confidentiality by refraining from disclosing private information to others except when it is necessary for the client's care or as expressly approved in writing. In doing so, the midwife must also look to the woman for guidance on sharing personal information with family members and friends who may be attending appointments, a birth, or some other aspect of the woman's care.

Healthcare professionals often find themselves in confidentiality dilemmas with family members. Typically, midwives encounter situations in which family members are present during exams or a birth. In these cases, the presence of the individual at the appointment or birth provides some level of implicit understanding that the observers are privy to the routine care provided in their presence; however, when information relating to lab work or medical history is at issue, the clinician should establish privacy with the client prior to discussing these details.

Information that is shared with family members should be limited to that which was approved by the client in advance with the client's best interests in mind. The woman and her partner control what information is shared with family and friends. Usually the midwife can discuss this with the client before the birth. Even when we become familiar with the family members of our clients, midwives maintain professionalism. In an emergency situation, providing critical care is primary, although the healthcare provider must remain mindful of maintaining privacy. For example, if a laboring woman is unable to communicate and you must look to a family member to make a decision about your client's health care, share only the information that is relevant to the situation. When sharing privacy information with family members, always consider the client's best interests.

What may appear to a clinician as general and benign information could be regarded as sensitive and private to a client. A midwife should not even disclose that a woman is in her care unless there is a clear indication that such information does not breach privacy. For example, if hired by a woman who was once under the care of a colleague, the midwife does not have the right to share this new relationship with her colleague. Midwives must turn to their clients for guidance about disclosures without making assumptions.

A healthcare professional should not discuss a client's information where others may overhear, even if a name is not used. Other details of care information may unintentionally identify the person to a bystander. Further, sharing case information in public places reflects poorly on healthcare professionals, and may even undermine trust in clinicians (Ives Erickson & Millar, 2005). This rule applies to emails, blogs, and case histories provided either in print or orally. Emails and faxes should include a privacy statement. Faxing of records requires a secure and private fax line. Midwives must be cognizant of the potential for confidentiality breaches when using the telephone, digital records, the Internet, and written correspondence. "The health care sector's overall shift to information digitization may prove to be one of the greatest challenges to privacy, confidentiality, and security" (Kumekawa, 2005, n.p.). Maintaining the privacy of healthcare records is further complicated by computerized patient records and managed care models (Aiken, 2009). Unless a client provides written permission to do so, midwives should not share birth stories or any aspect of their clients' histories in public places, electronic or otherwise.

When consulting, collaborating, or transferring care, sharing a client's private information may be essential for the quality of her care. Include a statement on collaboration of care in your privacy policy. Inform clients before collaborating or consulting with other professionals. Inform your clients of your policy for sharing information when transferring care. Obtain written consent, when possible, prior to initiating collaborative care or transferring care to another provider. Obscure identifying information unless the recipient of records is directly involved in the client's care. Clearly communicating with clients about the dissemination of their private records facilitates client control of records and promotes autonomy.

Confidentiality in Other Relationships

We have a duty to maintain confidentiality to nonclients as well. These may include colleagues, students, other professionals, and individuals who are "client-like" (see Chapter 5, "Who Is the Client?"). Jones (2000) describes a clinical situation in which the father of the baby confides to the midwife his probable intention of divorcing his wife when explaining his aversion to a vasectomy. "The consequences of violating such confidences, from the viewpoint of the families concerned, would be devastating and, as professionals, we must not help to create such an outcome" (p. 63). Similarly, negative consequences could arise should a midwife disclose personal information about a colleague. For example, a midwife who discloses the sexual orientation of another midwife could jeopardize the latter's safety or employment. When professionals collaborate, they have the responsibility to maintain the privacy of those involved.

Confidentiality in Peer Review

Peer review is a special context for sharing details of client information, yet steps must be taken to protect the identity of the client and rules must be set for participants to keep shared information strictly private. When charts are shared at a peer review, all identifying information should be obscured, including names, family members' names, and addresses. Other identifying information, such as age, parity, and birth setting, may be shared if it is relevant to the peer review process. Extraneous information should be obscured in an effort to minimize the chances of a client being identified by a participant in the peer review. Likewise, a clinician should avoid sharing similar information in verbal reports to peers. If one suspects a relationship between a participant in the peer review and the client, ethics may require the clinician to avoid presenting the chart. Vigilance is required to protect the client's privacy during a peer review. Helpful guidelines for peer review, including instructions regarding confidentiality, are available from the North American Registry of Midwives (NARM, 2006).

CASE EXAMPLES

CASE 1

Casey, a certified nurse–midwife (CNM) working for a small community hospital in her hometown, has recently been trained on the new electronic records system. As a practitioner, she now has access to all of the hospital's active files. This has changed her manner of collecting histories from her clients because of her awareness of other people's access to her clients' records. Departing from her previous system, she does not report current or past drug use, and she lists therapeutic abortions as spontaneous. Casey omits data that she feels could harm her clients.

Questions

1. Are Casey's actions legitimate means to protect her clients' privacy?
2. What potential harm could result from Casey's actions?
3. When weighing values of privacy against those of policy, on which side should a clinician err?

Analysis

In a small, rural environment, a clinician is often challenged by issues of privacy and confidentiality. A midwife may be involved with the maternity care of a significant portion of the population, and she will be in confidence with both current and past clients. To protect a client's privacy, a rural midwife may be compelled to withhold from colleagues information and records that she deems unnecessary for her client's care. In doing so, the clinician must weigh the risks and benefits of sharing and recording information.

Thus, the midwife balances two ethical principles: do no harm and confidentiality. As the New Zealand College of Midwives' Philosophy and Code of Ethics (n.d.) states, "[M]idwives have a responsibility to ensure that no action or omission on their part places the woman at risk" (n.p.). A midwife who wishes to protect a client from dissemination of aspects of her personal history must also be mindful of the responsibility to avoid omission of essential aspects of the client's medical history. Thus, ethical care requires a balancing of disclosure and nondisclosure with the client's best interests in mind.

The context of the care is an important consideration in making confidentiality decisions. If a rural hospital employs relatives of a client, and these employees also have access to records, a clinician has reason to pause regarding privacy. Only the information that is necessary for optimal health care should be recorded, whereas information that may be harmful to a client should be protected.

If a woman reports to her midwife that she has been the victim of domestic violence, and her spouse has relatives employed at the hospital, making this information accessible to those employees could present a danger to the client. Yet, if the clinician omits this important information and her client arrives in the emergency room with a broken arm, the doctor who sees her may not have information that would lead to suspicions of abuse, which might lead to further harm if the woman were to return to the abusive spouse without appropriate counseling.

Each situation should be scrutinized individually. Casey's practice of never recording drug use and abortions may not be the best way to serve all of her clients. If a client with an addiction continues to use teratogenic drugs during pregnancy, and Casey had failed to report her prior drug use, Casey may be considered at fault should there be a bad outcome. Rather than routine omission of potentially relevant information, Casey should exercise caution in recording potentially volatile information that could affect a client's care while avoiding reporting extraneous information. In some cases, allowing the client to make determinations about the sharing of her private data may be the best course of action.

With knowledge that others may have access to private information, a client may decide to censor what is shared with the midwife. To facilitate intimacy in the relationship and promote woman-centered care, the midwife and client can discuss what information should be included in the record. The midwife should set necessary boundaries to reflect ethical practices while acknowledging that some content may not be necessary to record.

There is no general rule that applies across the board in relation to privacy. We have guidelines to help us make decisions, but it is up to us as clinicians to exercise our best judgment when sharing privacy information. Electronic record systems that allow broad access to patient records come at a price. It is up to those of us who are given confidential information to choose wisely how to guard it.

CASE 2

A midwife refers a client to a physician for a diagnostic ultrasound. In response to a request for records from the doctor's office, the midwife faxes over the client's entire prenatal record. This information includes the client's history, prenatal flow sheet, and lab work. When the client arrives at her next appointment with the midwife, she is upset because the doctor had questioned her about her sexual orientation, lecturing her on his views regarding the limitations of a lesbian couple's ability to raise healthy children.

Questions

1. What caution should be used when sharing information regarding sexual orientation?

2. What considerations are relevant to faxing client records?
3. How can the midwife inform a client of how information is shared with other clinicians?

Analysis

Information should be shared on a need-to-know basis (Ives Erickson & Millar, 2005). If a client requires a diagnostic ultrasound from a physician, the physician does not need to know the client's sexual orientation to do his or her job. Likewise, other information in the history may be unnecessary for this physician to access. The midwife should only send information that is necessary to facilitate care. Usually, information needed for a sonogram is limited to last menstrual period and the client's personal identity and contact information. Sometimes, insurance information is required to secure an appointment. If additional information is requested, the midwife should consider the necessity of that information for the client's care prior to sharing it with another clinician.

Clinicians should exercise caution when sharing information regarding a client's sexual orientation. Sexual orientation involves the right to privacy, a right that has been upheld by the U.S. Supreme Court in *Lawrence v. Texas* (2003). In general, one should not divulge another person's sexual orientation without permission to do so. In a clinical relationship, this general social rule is even more important. There have been numerous cases of violence relating to membership in a sexual minority group, and family and community discord is an all-too-common experience for lesbian and gay couples. Adding stress to the lives of people seeking maternity care by "outing" them to others does them a great disservice.

Setting up a method of communicating your privacy policies to your clients is an important aspect of building a clinical relationship. Clients should be informed in advance if you are sharing their records with others; this can be communicated through a document that the client signs at the onset of care. Within this document, a midwife should list ways in which a client's record may be shared, including with the private insurer, collaborating healthcare providers, during peer review, and among office coworkers, including nurses and receptionists. You may include methods of transmitting documents, including electronic records, to ensure that your client has a clear understanding of how her record may be shared and the possibility of others accessing her private file.

Faxing records to other offices and clinics always increases the chance of breaching confidentiality. It is imperative that faxes have a secure line and that the receiver has a private fax machine. Public faxing is discouraged, with few exceptions, because it expands access to private records. For example, if a fax line is shared by both a doctor's office and a health spa, the health spa employees also have access to faxes sent to the doctor's office. If a midwife is aware of an insecure fax line or of expanded access to faxes, it behooves her to send the file by mail or to deliver it by courier.

This case scenario illustrates the importance of confidentiality in the midwife-client relationship. Because private information was provided to an outsider without consent, the relationship has been jeopardized. Forgiveness for an oversight like this one is possible, and likely warranted, but the clinician should take steps to avoid another case of confidentiality encroachment by reviewing information prior to sharing it with other providers, and omitting information that is irrelevant to their role in caring for the woman.

CASE 3

A community of midwives comes together biannually for peer review. Shelly, a homebirth midwife in private practice, brings a case history of a client who transferred out of her care due to mental illness. The client had had no prior prenatal care and sought a midwife for a home birth. The client reported a prior diagnosis of bipolar disorder during the initial interview. By the third prenatal visit, the midwife questioned the woman's mental health and associated risk factors, including the safety of home birth.

As she is presenting her case to the group, another midwife, Margaret, begins to suspect that she knows the identity of the woman in the case. She becomes uncomfortable with the situation as the client's behavior is described. After transferring out of Shelly's care, the client gave birth at the hospital where Margaret works. In this capacity, Margaret had heard another side of the story from the client. Based on this report, Margaret felt that Shelly had abandoned the client. She sat quietly as other midwives commented on aspects of the case and offered feedback.

Finally, Margaret chimed in, unable to withhold her own emotions. Her criticism of the homebirth midwife was unduly harsh. She knew that she shouldn't divulge her relationship with the client at hand, so she focused instead on Shelly's lack of sensitivity to mental illness and subsequent potential harm. Shelly took the criticism as a personal attack and left the peer review early, leaving Margaret angry and stunned.

Questions

1. How could this situation have been avoided?
2. Who is the victim in this scenario?
3. What guidelines should be agreed upon and enforced in a peer review?

Analysis

Peer reviews present risks for clinicians regarding the maintenance of confidentiality. Often, paper charts are copied and distributed with names and identifying information obscured. The purpose of peer review is to provide learning opportunities for midwives in a geographical area by allowing them to monitor one another's practices. To achieve this purpose, only aspects of the chart that are relevant to the case study should be shared.

If an intrapartum complication arises, portions of the prenatal record may or may not be appropriate to share for a peer review. If there were possible indications during the pregnancy that relate to the intrapartum complication, then providing a copy of the prenatal record is warranted. However, if adequate analysis of the case can be made with just the intrapartum record, then other contents of the file should be omitted from the peer review. Only information that is applicable to the situation regarding the complication of the case should be shared with others in a peer review.

Shelly may have shared more information than was appropriate for the case at hand, which may have led Margaret to make connections between Shelly's client and the woman whose birth she attended. There is not enough information to make this assessment, but confidentiality should always be a primary goal of a peer review.

Margaret acted inappropriately by listening through the entire case review even when she had established that she had identified Shelly's client. Margaret could have done one of two things to avoid damage to the client's confidentiality. She could have interrupted Shelly's case presentation and stated that she thought that she might know the woman in the scenario, without sharing any other information regarding the nature of their relationship. Alternatively, Margaret could have excused herself immediately, once she realized that she had a relationship with Shelly's client. To allow yourself access to private information that is assumed to be confidential is a breach of confidentiality, even when you are not the care provider directly involved in the case.

Although both midwives in Case 3 were stressed by the situation, the only victim of the situation is the client. Unbeknownst to her, a midwife at her birth now has access to her prior midwife's record of her care. This may change the nature of their relationship, and may present challenges should the woman seek midwifery care in the future from either of the midwives in this scenario.

Peer review must undergo the scrutiny of ethics so that the client's right to privacy and dignity are upheld at all times. In birthing communities, the possibility always exists of a woman being in the care of a midwife who has heard a peer review of one of her previous births from another midwife. Even in a large urban setting, case studies should always assume that this is a possibility and protect a woman's identity from inadvertently being disclosed.

Setting up guidelines for peer review that include steps to protect confidentiality is essential. These steps should include basic actions to avoid the use of names or other identifying information and to limit the information shared to that which is necessary for case evaluation. Further, attendees at a peer review should agree to either leave the room if they suspect that they know the identity of a client in a case scenario or interrupt the presenter with that information before harm is done. These steps will go far toward avoiding unintended breaches of confidentiality in a setting that is supposed to maintain the highest of professional standards—the peer review.

REFERENCES

Aiken, T. D. (2009). *Legal and ethical issues in health occupations* (2nd ed.). New Orleans, LA: Elsevier.

American College of Nurse-Midwives (ACNM). (2004). *Code of ethics of the American College of Nurse-Midwives.* Silver Spring, MD: Author.

Griswold v. Connecticut, 381 U.S. 479 (1965).

Health Insurance Portability and Accountability Act (HIPAA). Pub. L. No. 104-191, 110 Stat. 1936 (1996).

Ives Erickson, J., & Millar, S. (2005). Caring for patients while respecting their privacy: Renewing our commitment. *Online Journal of Issues in Nursing, 10*(2). Retrieved December 15, 2008, from MEDLINE with Full Text database.

Jones, S. R. (2000). *Ethics in midwifery.* London: Harcourt.

Kumekawa, J. (2005, May). Overview and summary: HIPAA—how our health care world has changed. *Online Journal of Issues in Nursing, 10*(2). Retrieved December 15, 2008, from CINAHL Plus with Full Text database.

Lawrence v. Texas, 539 U.S. 558 (2003).

North American Registry of Midwives (NARM). (2006). *NARM community peer review: Community peer review process.* Retrieved August 2, 2009, from http://www.narm.org/peerreview.htm

New Zealand College of Midwives. (n.d.). *Philosophy and code of ethics.* Retrieved February 2, 2009, from www.midwife.org.nz/index.cfm/1,179.html

Privacy Act, 5 U.S.C. § 552a (1974).

Rothman, B. K. (1979). *Two models in maternity care: Defining and negotiating reality.* New York: New York University Press.

Tschudin, V. (2003). *Ethics in nursing: The caring relationship.* London: Elsevier.

United Nations (UN). (1948). *The Universal Declaration of Human Rights.* Retrieved December 8, 2008, from http://www.un.org/Overview/rights.html

U.S. Department of Health and Human Services. (n.d.) *Health insurance privacy: The Health Insurance Portability and Accountability Act of 1996.* Retrieved September 16, 2009, from http://www.hhs.gov/ocr/privacy

CHAPTER 4

Informed Consent and Choice

INFORMED CONSENT

Midwives respect their clients' autonomy and right to make decisions for themselves (American College of Nurse-Midwives [ACNM], 2004; National Association of Certified Professional Midwives [NACPM], 2004). Although this concept is fairly straightforward, the application of consent becomes complicated in practice (Lützén, 1997). This chapter introduces the concept of informed consent and choice and highlights some of the ethical challenges associated with midwife-client consent practices.

Many readers have experience with informed consent[1] from their relationships with doctors or researchers. For example, a physician asks for your informed consent before initiating a surgical procedure, and a psychologist seeks your informed consent before starting psychotherapy. If you have been a participant in a research study, the investigator most likely sought your informed consent to participate in the study. Just as doctors, psychologists, and researchers seek consent, so do midwives.

We want to ensure that midwifery clients understand our services before consenting to care. Our experience as patients, practitioners, researchers, and research participants has been that in practice, informed consent is often not properly obtained. Failure to obtain informed consent represents a serious breach in ethical responsibilities and must not be taken lightly. What follows is a thorough discussion of the critical components of informed consent.

To ensure that clients are treated ethically, midwives must obtain informed consent before initiating services. There are three essential components to in formed consent: clients must be *knowing*, *competent*, and must consent *voluntarily*. Each of these components merits discussion.

---

[1]Many midwives prefer the term *informed choice* over *informed consent*. Because most of the literature in ethics uses the latter, we begin with this convention but later introduce the former.

Knowing

A client should be given enough information to make a good choice for herself before consenting to services. The element of "knowing" is what differentiates mere consent from *informed* consent. Clients must be informed of potential benefits, risks, likely outcomes, and alternatives so that they can make an informed choice. To bring this concept to life, suppose your doctor recommends a surgical procedure and asks for your consent. You would want to know exactly what the procedure would involve, how long it would take, how the procedure might help you, the likelihood that the surgery would be successful, and how much it would cost. You would also want to know about potential side effects and the likelihood of experiencing those side effects, whether there were alternative procedures that could give you the same results, or how well you would fare if you elected to not have the procedure. The physician would need to provide you with all this information so that you could make an informed choice.

This example illustrates how much information a professional must share with a client about a specific procedure. As professional midwives, we are ethically bound to provide comprehensive information to clients about procedures so that clients can make informed choices. However, clients must be informed not only about specific procedures, but also about consenting to receive care from a midwife. When a potential client seeks the care of a midwife, the midwife has an ethical obligation to provide the potential client with sufficient information so that the client can make an informed decision. Moreover, this information must be provided in a format that is easily understood by the client. Technical jargon should be avoided, and information must be provided in the potential client's native language.

Some states may have laws that outline the specific information that must be provided to potential clients. Because state legal requirements vary, it will be important for you to be fully aware of the informed consent requirements in your state (your state midwifery association is a good resource). This book considers the ethical requirements rather than legal mandates. Consequently, you may find that ethics requires more of you than the law. We encourage midwives to go beyond what is required by law so that ethical standards are maintained.

The midwife who is consulting with a prospective client is *ethically* bound to provide the following information:

- Training and education (e.g., the midwife's level of formal education, such as university and/or midwifery training programs; apprenticeships, etc.)
- Credentials/licensure (e.g., CNM, CPM, CM, LM, DEM, traditional midwife)
- Legal status of midwifery in your state
- Continuing education (e.g., hours per year, currency)

- Experience (e.g., years in practice)
- Cost of services
- Services provided
- Additional services not included in base fee
- Scope of practice
- Payment options (e.g., method of payment, insurance, payment plans, barter, policy for failure to pay)
- Potential benefits and risk
- Alternatives to midwifery care
- Emergency care plan
- Policies, procedures, and protocols
- Statistics for transports, cesarean sections, and other outcomes

Providing this much information to a potential client may seem overwhelming, particularly given the need to ensure that the client not only receives the information but also understands it. Consequently, the informed consent process takes time and should never be hurried. Note that many clients may not understand the acronyms, jargon, and technical language of midwifery, and that terms such as "CNM" or "ruptured membranes" must be explained. A midwife can concisely provide the information that a potential client would need to consent to care through the use of an easy-to-read handout or standardized verbal explanation in conjunction with a written consent form.

Clients and potential clients should be encouraged to ask questions, take time to think about their options, and seek additional information on their own before consenting to services or procedures. Some situations in midwifery practice do not afford the luxury of time to ponder options (e.g., emergency transport in labor from home birth to hospital). Such situations are discussed later in this chapter.

Competent

Before we provide services to others, we are ethically obligated to ensure that the person consenting is competent to do so. Competency takes on a number of meanings in the context of informed consent. For example, in most states, individuals must be 18 years old (or legally designated as emancipated minors) to be considered competent to give consent. We find this age requirement to be somewhat arbitrary, given the wide range of developmental maturity in the teen and early adult years. Some 17-year-olds are more mature than some 19-year-olds. Nevertheless, tradition has held that competency to give consent begins on one's 18th birthday.

Many states have exceptions to the traditional 18-year-old cutoff when a minor becomes pregnant. In such states, the pregnant minor is legally "emancipated" and therefore legally able to consent for herself. However, we must distinguish the legal requirements for consent from the ethical requirements for consent. Even if a 15-year-old pregnant adolescent is *legally* considered competent to consent for herself, to be ethical a midwife must assess the degree to which such a client is cognitively and emotionally competent to provide her informed consent.

How does a midwife obtain informed consent from a 17-year-old client? In most helping professions (e.g., psychology, social work, counseling), the protocol is to obtain informed consent from the minor client's parent or guardian and to obtain informed *assent* from the minor client. *Assent* is simply the consent term used for minors. One potential problem of seeking parental consent as well as the minor's assent is that the parent and minor may disagree. We believe that midwives should not provide services to individuals who do not want those services, because this is a clear violation of client autonomy. Therefore, providing midwifery care to a minor without her assent (i.e., involuntarily) would be unethical. Providing services to a minor without her parent's consent could become a legal liability for the midwife and potentially disrupt family relationships. Midwives are advised to proceed with caution and help the family achieve harmony and collaboration regarding the pregnancy.

Another facet of the "competency" element of informed consent concerns the client's cognitive ability. Individuals with intellectual and developmental disabilities may be deemed incompetent to consent for themselves, largely because they may have difficulty understanding and processing the information provided to them. In many such cases, a competent individual has been given power of attorney to make such decisions. Midwives have an ethical responsibility to ensure that potential clients are competent to consent for themselves or, if they are not competent, that a competent individual can consent for them.

Voluntary

Informed consent should never be obtained by coercion or against someone's will. The thought of forcing someone to consent to midwifery services may be unthinkable to many readers (picture the midwife threatening the pregnant woman to consent *or else!*), but the voluntary nature of informed consent becomes relevant in more subtle ways. Pressures to consent to services, treatments, or procedures may be unintentional but powerful influences on clients' decision making. For example, the midwife who discourages the client from investigating alternatives to the recommended procedure may be pressuring the client to consent and thereby diminishing the extent to which the informed consent is voluntary.

The voluntary nature of consent may also be threatened if the midwife appeals to clients' fears when requesting consent. In fact, some research has demonstrated that fear interferes with problem-solving skills and may result in behaviors directed at avoiding crisis (Lerner & Keltner, 2000; Smith & Lazarus, 1993). In such a state, clients may not feel that they can consent voluntarily. For example, if a midwife tells a client that failure to comply with a recommended protocol could result in negative outcomes, the client's ability to make an informed choice could be impaired by the fears aroused. This is not to suggest that midwives should withhold information that is potentially frightening. Rather, we emphasize the importance of providing balanced information that accurately represents the potential risks and benefits of choices. Providing selective information geared toward scaring the client into consenting is inherently unethical, because it undermines the client's ability to voluntarily consent.

The Code of Ethics of the American College of Nurse-Midwives (ACNM, 2004; see Appendix C) identifies a number of factors that could potentially constrain a woman's freedom to voluntarily consent. These include the following:

- Undue influence of family members
- Undue influence of the midwife or other professionals
- Financial limitations
- Lack of privacy when receiving information about options
- Limited access to alternative procedures or practitioners
- Abusive relationships

Given the potential limitations on a woman's ability to freely make choices about her pregnancy and birth, midwives have a responsibility to proactively promote voluntary consent. We can promote voluntary consent by attending to situational factors, such as those listed above, that could potentially interfere with a woman's ability to freely consent. For example, by empowering clients with information to make good decisions for themselves rather than using our influence to shape their decisions, we encourage voluntary consent. Another way that midwives can address these concerns is by ensuring privacy.

Midwives have an ethical obligation to protect the privacy of the women they serve. Chapter 3 provided a comprehensive discussion of the related issues of privacy and confidentiality, but we want to emphasize the relationship between privacy and informed consent here. As mentioned earlier, lack of privacy may interfere with a woman's ability to freely consent to services or procedures. Midwives "provide an environment where privacy is protected and in which all pertinent information is shared without bias, coercion, or deception" (ACNM, 2004, p. 9). Without a doubt, the data provided to a woman so that she can make an informed choice must be without bias. But how does privacy interact with information? A midwife could feel limited regarding the amount of information that she could share with a woman in the presence of family members and friends. In such cases, the midwife should ensure that informed consent is obtained in a private setting.

Withdrawing Consent

When a client provides her informed consent for midwifery care and services, she maintains her right to withdraw her consent at any time. Consenting to midwifery care does not "lock in" the client; she can choose to discontinue services or refuse particular aspects of care. In fact, potential clients should be informed at the outset that should they consent to services, they have the right to withdraw their consent at any time. This is particularly relevant because clients' life circumstances change over time. For example, suppose a client consents to midwifery services but later learns that her health insurance does not reimburse for midwifery services. She may elect to withdraw her consent and seek care from a provider who is covered under her health insurance plan. A client who hires a midwife and later discovers that she is pregnant with twins may also decide to withdraw consent if she feels safer birthing with a physician.

A PROCESS ORIENTATION TO INFORMED CONSENT

What's the difference between an event and a process? For some, leaving the house is an event; walking out the door. For parents of infants and toddlers, leaving the house is a process; getting on socks and shoes, filling a diaper bag, loading the stroller, and packing a snack. These activities are all part of the *process* of leaving. Although many treat informed consent as an event (e.g., "sign here"), we advocate for a process orientation. To do so, we contrast conventional blanket consent with a process orientation.

Blanket Consent

Blanket consent refers to the process of obtaining a client's consent for any and all potential services at the beginning of care. This might be accomplished by providing the potential client with a consent document that lists the services that will or could be provided and states that by signing the document, the client gives consent to all such services in advance. Such blanket consent is unethical and should not be used. The ethical problems with blanket consent are many, but the most pervasive concern can be found in the fact that a client cannot make informed decisions at the outset about unforeseen issues that may arise. The client who gives blanket consent at the initiation of services may be subjected to interventions at a later date that make her uncomfortable. Alternatively, a midwife should obtain informed consent on an ongoing basis.

A midwife's protocol for a given complication does not function implicitly as voluntary informed consent. Rather, a protocol must be disclosed to a client at an appropriate time and with adequate explanation. If a midwife transfers care of all breech births to a physician, she has an obligation to disclose this information to a client with a suspected breech presentation as early as possible. This provides the client with time to consider the risks and benefits of such a protocol and to research the physician's track record for vaginal breech births, if she so desires. Other protocols and policies that are likely to affect a significant proportion of a midwife's clients should be stated routinely at consultation or the onset of care. These protocols may include criteria for antepartum, intrapartum, and postpartum transfer of care. Certain complications that arise during intrapartum care do not permit time for disclosure. Still, every effort should be made by the midwife to ensure that consent is voluntary for each procedure.

Informed Consent as a Process

An alternative to blanket consent involves treating informed consent as a process, which is well established in other fields such as psychology (Gottlieb, 1997; Lasser & Klose, 2007; Pope & Vasquez, 1991). Unfortunately, many healthcare providers treat informed consent as a one-shot event: sign here to consent to treatment, whatever that may be. This is generally regarded as unethical because the act of obtaining consent for a wide range of services does not account for the significant changes that almost always occur over time. Moreover, midwives cannot possibly inform clients about all of the potential risks and benefits of every potential complication, procedure, or decision. Therefore, we reject blanket consent as an unethical practice and promote informed consent as a process.

When midwives employ a process orientation to informed consent, they begin with an initial consent to receive services that is both written and oral. Over the course of treatment, the midwife revisits informed consent as needed to ensure that the client has opportunities to take an active role in making informed choices about her care. Situations that might call for additional informed consent include but are not limited to, the following:

- Vaginal exams
- Palpation
- Holding back cervical lip
- Putting the client on oxygen
- Running blood panels
- Administration of medications
- Episiotomy
- Cesarean section
- Transport to a hospital from a home birth
- Transfer of care to a physician
- Putting in an IV
- Fundal massage
- Breech presentation
- Twins
- Amniotomy

SOME LOGISTICAL CONSIDERATIONS

As mentioned earlier, informed consent must be documented in writing. A signed and written consent form serves several purposes. First, it documents that the midwife provided sufficient information to the client so that she could make an informed choice, and the signature documents the client's consent. Second, a written consent form greatly minimizes miscommunication (e.g., "You never told me that you don't attend breech births!"). Finally, written consent forms give clients an opportunity to spend time thinking about their decision. They can take the consent form home, read and reread it, show it to friends and relatives, and then make a thoughtful, informed decision without feeling pressured. Clients should be given a copy of the consent form to keep for their records.

Consent forms must be easily understood by clients. Therefore, midwives must create or use documents that are in the client's native language and written at the client's reading level. Because the average adult literacy level in the United States falls within an eighth- to ninth-grade reading level (Kirsch, Jungeblut, Jenkins, & Kolstad, 1993), midwives should make an effort to assess the reading level of consent forms used and adjust it as needed. Readability also requires minimizing jargon and, when needed, explaining terminology that is not commonly used by the general public.

We have provided guidelines for informed consent/choice documents published by the North American Registry of Midwives (NARM, 2008) at the end of this chapter. What follows is a consent form checklist that can be used to help you develop your own consent form:

- ☐ Eighth- to ninth-grade reading level
- ☐ Written in client's native language
- ☐ Includes statement that consent is voluntary
- ☐ Includes statement that consent can be withdrawn at any point in time
- ☐ When appropriate, differentiates assent and consent
- ☐ Copy of form is provided to client
- ☐ Provides a summary of potential risks and benefits

When informed consent is applied as a process, midwives and clients experience this important ethical standard as more than simply a document. Moving past the piece of paper by making informed consent an ongoing dialogue has the potential to enhance the midwife-client relationship, erode power differentials, empower clients, and increase client satisfaction. The benefits of this approach cannot be overstated.

Informed consent as a process works best when midwives and clients communicate with each other frequently and effectively. Clients should be encouraged to ask questions about their care and treatment regularly and to communicate with midwives about changes in their health status. Midwives should listen closely to client concerns and questions and be diligent about documenting communications with clients.

Informed Consent Versus Informed Choice

Whereas many healthcare providers refer to *informed consent* in their ethical guidelines, most professional midwifery organizations have elected to use *informed choice* (ACNM, 2004; International Confederation of Midwives, 2003; Midwives Alliance of North America, 1997). Although the distinction may be subtle, we think that it is significant and reflects the values inherent in the Midwives Model of Care (MMOC) (Rothman, 1979). For example, the ACNM clearly goes beyond what it required for informed consent by noting that midwives "develop a partnership with the woman in which each shares relevant information that leads to informed decision making, consent to an evolving plan of care, and acceptance of responsibility for the outcome of their choices" (ACNM, 2004, p. 6). Whereas a traditional informed consent model conceptualizes the flow of information as going from the practitioner to the client, the ACNM guidelines view the sharing of information as bidirectional with the purpose being collaboration and shared responsibility.

The idea of shared responsibility deviates from the conventional medical model. Embedded in a culture of rampant litigation and blame, healthcare providers have spent fortunes on medical malpractice insurance as a shield against potential lawsuits. Undoubtedly, some of these suits have merit and irresponsible practitioners should be held liable. However, a significant fraction of claimants have failed to take responsibility for the choices they have made regarding their health care. Granted, many of them were likely offered a pro forma opportunity to merely consent (as opposed to giving truly *informed* consent), but the model perpetuates the notion of patients who are not at all responsible for their health care. Midwives offer an alternative paradigm: informed choice and shared responsibility in which women and their providers collaborate, exchange information freely, and share in the goals and responsibilities of care.

CASE EXAMPLES

CASE 1

Brandi is a 26-year-old who has had the benefits of midwifery care during her pregnancy. She arrives at her midwife's birth center in active labor. An initial exam shows a cervix that is 5cm dilated and 80% effaced. She is admitted to the birth center and her labor continues to progress. Two hours later, a second exam shows Brandi's cervix to be 6cm dilated and rigid. There are no complications with the mother or fetus, but the midwife expresses a need to rupture membranes to assist the labor progression. Brandi isn't quite sure what that means, but agrees that progressing labor is certainly desirable. The midwife uses an amniohook to perform AROM (artificial rupture of membranes).

An asynclitic head is noted immediately after the procedure. The midwife then suggests that she adjust the baby's head internally so that it is well applied to the cervix and labor can progress. Brandi agrees that labor progressing is generally desirable, and she allows the midwife to manually rotate the baby's head. This procedure is very uncomfortable for Brandi, and it takes a total of three contraction cycles to complete. During this time, the fetal heart rate becomes slightly tachycardic and the mother sobs. The birth proceeds normally after a few minutes of calming and maternal position change. After the birth, the mother expresses concern over the procedures that occurred, their necessity and potential side effects. She feels dissatisfied with her midwife's explanations of the procedures during labor and expresses her feelings at a postpartum appointment.

Questions

1. Did the midwife receive informed consent from her client for each of the procedures?
2. Does the midwife have an obligation to disclose the potential risks and benefits of each procedure she uses?
3. If this were an emergency situation, how would informed consent be handled?

Analysis

Brandi's midwife behaved as many obstetricians and midwives do in similar situations. She briefly discussed her rationale for optional procedures with the client before undertaking them. She carried out the procedures, we assume, skillfully, and checked for the effects of the procedures on the mother and baby, following up as needed. Fortunately, the procedures seem to have had the desired effect of progressing labor. The baby was born without complication. Yet, the mother is dissatisfied.

A mother's dissatisfaction may be out of her midwife's control, yet her clients' understanding of procedures is something that the midwife can take action to improve. Although typical, this mother's case was handled poorly. The limited information offered to the client failed to cover risks, benefits, alternatives, the possibility of waiting, and the effects of doing nothing.

Two common informed choice education tools have the acronyms BRAND and BRAIN. BRAND stands for benefits, risks, alternatives, now-or-later, and decision. It is the caregiver's role to cover this information with clients prior to a procedure such as AROM. Similarly, BRAIN outlines benefits, risks, alternatives, intuition, and [doing] nothing. The midwife in Case 1 did mention the benefits of progressing labor for both procedures, but she failed to inform the client of the potential risks of either procedure. Nor did she give alternatives to either procedure, such as ambulation for asynclitism. She did not discuss the necessity of the timing, or lack thereof, of either procedure. "Intuition," mentioned in the BRAIN acronym, calls for the midwife to ask the client's feelings about a procedure to get a sense of her position emotionally; "nothing," also in BRAIN, refers to the potential outcome of not doing the procedure or any alternatives. "Nothing" is the expected outcome if the midwife does not intervene.

It is questionable whether each and every procedure requires the process of BRAIN or BRAND, but a clinician who is practiced in informed consent can help a client to easily navigate the informed consent process. For example, Brandi's midwife could have said, "Your cervix is dilated to 6cm. It hasn't progressed much since you came in here a couple of hours ago, and it has a rigidity to it that may hold the dilation here for a while unless we change something. Usually, I advise rupturing membranes in cases like yours, but I could massage it a bit during the next contraction to see if it will relax and stretch. Alternatively, we could just wait and see if it progresses on its own, as it may if you move around a bit and the baby rotates and descends into the pelvis. How do you feel about these choices?" This explanation opens up the situation to discussion and allows the client an active role in the management of her birth. Once given the choice, if the client chooses AROM, the midwife should cover potential risks: "Artificial rupture of membranes increases risk of infection; it will likely make contractions stronger; if the head is not well applied to the cervix, it is possible for a loop of cord to come down and cause fetal distress." Regardless of her choices, the client is likely to be more satisfied with the situation because she has played an active and informed role in her care management.

If the baby in this scenario were distressed, the midwife would attempt to give the client informed consent prior to undertaking further intervention. The care provider has an obligation to attempt to obtain informed consent for procedures in emergency situations. Yet, contextual factors, such as time, a woman's cognitive state, and the need for immediate intervention may limit the provider's abilities to obtain consent.

CASE 2

Shannon is a 35-year-old client who is 41 weeks pregnant with her fifth baby when she goes into labor. Her midwife arrives at her house and begins monitoring the labor, while another midwife accompanies her to the birth to assist with the delivery. The labor progresses quickly and the membranes rupture at the beginning of the second stage, after which the baby's head descends rapidly into a crown. With the next contraction, the head is born, but the midwives notice that it doesn't rotate and a turtle sign is noted, followed by a rapid darkening in the baby's skin color. The primary midwife speaks directly to her client: "Shannon, the baby needs help getting out. I need you to follow my directions carefully and stay calm." The second midwife then follows the lead of the primary midwife, in preparation for a McRoberts maneuver and suprapubic pressure. "We need to put you on your back with your legs way back, Shannon. Hold your legs like this. I'm going to have to put my hands inside of you to rotate the baby. Please focus on your breathing while I do this." Shannon cooperates beautifully and the midwives are able to successfully deliver a 10-pound baby. After the delivery, the primary midwife explains the shoulder dystocia to Shannon, including the need to act quickly. At a later postpartum visit, the midwife invites questions about the birth and the procedures used to assist with the delivery. Shannon expresses gratitude at having the opportunity to review the birth and asks a couple of questions. The midwife discloses more details about the shoulder dystocia and leaves the conversation open to future discussion.

Questions

1. Did the midwife behave ethically during the delivery?
2. How did contextual factors shape the midwife's ability to obtain informed consent?
3. Is there anything that the midwives could have said or done differently that would have facilitated informed consent at this birth?
4. What is the midwife's ethical obligation after a birth like this, when an invasive procedure is undertaken without informed consent?

Analysis

Shannon's baby was born healthy due to the skills and cooperation of all parties. Many midwives would agree that the desired outcome trumps all, and that there is no need to revisit this birth. Yet, consent was breached in this situation because the emergency at hand did not permit adequate opportunity to obtain it. Therefore, it is the responsibility of the midwife to revisit the birth with the client and explain the necessity of acting quickly without discussion, allowing the client an opportunity to respond and pose questions. Informed consent is not retroactive, however, and a clinician's debriefing with a client after an invasive procedure serves solely to educate and empower the client with information related to the care received.

Some emergency situations do not permit opportunities for informed consent, but it should be sought whenever possible. When there is time to explain the risks and benefits of a procedure, such as a cesarean section, the care provider is ethically bound to provide the client with informed consent. It is inadequate for a care provider to simply state his or her rationale for a procedure, as demonstrated in Case 1. When a client agrees to a clinician's rationale for surgery, for instance, she is consenting, but without informed consent. This is often the tactic that health professionals use to persuade a client to agree to procedures when a complication arises. When contextual factors, such as time, allow for informed consent, an emergency situation does not preclude a clinician from his or her responsibility in obtaining it.

CASE 3

Selina is a 19-year-old primigravida. She received prenatal care at a clinic connected to a hospital that employs midwives. She is in her 37th week of pregnancy with premature rupture of membranes (PROM) when she arrives at the hospital. Her primary language is Spanish, but her husband speaks fluent English and accompanies her to labor and delivery. A midwife and nurse meet Selina and her spouse in her hospital room. The midwife confirms ruptured membranes and assists the nurse in admitting the client. The nurse speaks English to Selina, taking a brief history and explaining hospital admission paperwork. The midwife notices that Selina appears to fail to comprehend the information and questions and that the husband answers the questions for her. The midwife interrupts the admission process and asks the nurse if a Spanish-speaking nurse or medical interpreter is on duty. The nurse is certain that nobody on duty speaks fluent Spanish. The midwife asks that the nurse slow down the admission process to allow for the woman to comprehend.

As the admission process proceeds, a stack of paperwork is offered for Selina to sign. "This one is for pain-relief and epidural; in case of c-section, sign here," and so on. The midwife begins to draw blood from the client during the intake, speaking directly to the husband about the blood tests and asking him to translate to his wife. After intake is complete, both nurse and midwife leave the room. The midwife returns shortly with Pitocin and explains to Selina and her husband about inducing labor with medication. "When your waters are ruptured, there is greater risk of infection, so we'll also give you antibiotics. This medicine is to help start your labor so that the baby will come." She attempts to keep things simple so that the young couple understands. Eventually, Selina is set up with a Pitocin induction and antibiotic therapy. When active labor begins, the nurse comes in to offer epidural to "ease her pain and let her rest." The woman and spouse nod, not knowing that they already consented to all of these procedures at admission or that they have a right to ask questions and refuse any treatment option.

Questions

1. How many of the elements of informed consent (knowing, voluntary, competent) are met in this case?
2. How does the hospital admission process undermine informed consent?
3. What specific recommendations would you give the midwife in this situation to increase her client's access to information and empower her to make informed decisions about her care?
4. If Selina were a minor, what other considerations would arise?

Analysis

Selina and her partner did not receive adequate information about their care to give informed consent. Partly due to a language barrier, their access to information about procedures was limited. The midwife in the case was correct in questioning the woman's comprehension of the admission process. "If a third party is involved in the translation, midwives need to assess the veracity of translation and the understanding of the woman" (ACNM, 2004, p. 10). Yet, some hospitals are ill-equipped to meet the cultural needs of a diverse population, as in this case where a bilingual nurse was not available. Inadequate information further resulted from the routine process of a hospital admission.

Hospital admission policies tend to minimize informed consent for their patients, and it is the clinician's role to educate and inform clients of their care modalities. Here, the MMOC contrasts with medical/technocratic models. The midwife may meet resistance from nurses, doctors, and staff when advocating for client education and empowerment. Hospital administrators are likely to pressure midwives to conform to hospital policies. This situation presents a role challenge to hospital midwives who must distinguish their professional priorities. A midwife with privileges at a community hospital may have the advantage of acting more independently in client education and care modalities, whereas a staff midwife may be restricted by employment terms from acting outside of hospital policy. Thankfully, midwives who work in hospital settings have opportunities to offer women who birth in hospitals—the majority of American women—choices in childbirth, the first step of which is providing informed consent. In Selina's case, the information provided was inadequate for her informed choice, and her childbearing experience was overshadowed by a system that did not adequately meet her needs.

One can argue that Selina's consent was not voluntary, as is the experience of many minority women seeking medical care. The cultural barrier of deference to authority can pressure a woman to accept any terms of her care if guided by an authority figure to do so. Similarly, Selina's youth is a variable that can affect the voluntary nature of consent. If Selina were under the legal age of consent, her midwife would still be ethically bound to provide informed consent. A guardian's consent alone is inadequate to meet the voluntary requirements of informed consent. Young women are less likely to feel comfortable challenging an authority figure than are mature women, so the care provider must take additional steps to inform the client of her rights and ensure that her consent is both informed and voluntary.

Whose responsibility is it to bridge cultural and age differences? The nurse and midwife both hold responsibility in this case. The MMOC calls midwives to individualize care. A midwife serving a diverse population is required to learn cultural competency for the ethnic groups reflected in her clinical population (see

Chapter 10). Both the hospital and the midwife have an obligation to provide material in Spanish whenever possible. A Spanish speaker should be on call or brought in from another department of the hospital to translate for this client. Awareness of the power dynamics of age assists the midwife-client relationship. The midwife should inform the young woman of her rights and encourage her to think about risks and benefits of procedures before consenting to them.

CASE 4

Melinda is a 25-year-old mother consulting with a midwife for the first time. It is clear that she is well educated about childbirth options and models of care. She requests data regarding the practitioner's professional status, statistics, and physician backup arrangements. She further inquires about references and typical birthing scenarios, and asks questions regarding professional philosophy and style. The woman expresses her desire for a hands-off water birth, a midwife who will support her choices and a clear emergency backup plan.

After Melinda hires the midwife, she continues to be inquisitive and involved in every level of her care. She researches each lab test, and refuses the group B strep screen and vitamin K for her newborn. The midwife works with Melinda through her myriad of questions related to her birth plan. The midwife wants to meet Melinda's desire for information, but also wants to balance her desire for control with the reality of the unpredictability of birth. At childbirth classes, the midwife describes possible reasons for transfer of care and the importance of trust and cooperation in the midwife-client relationship.

At her birth, Melinda refuses to be checked for cervical dilation except when she is ready to push. The midwife is concerned about the baby's position and expresses the risks and benefits of doing a pelvic exam. Melinda continues to refuse the exam, and everything proceeds normally until variable decelerations are noted. The midwife explains to Melinda the need for a maternal position change to assist the baby. At her urging, Melinda ambulates around the room and settles into a forward-leaning position. The decelerations are no longer detectable. Again, the midwife suggests an exam to ensure that the baby's head is properly engaged, but Melinda continues to refuse.

Questions

1. How does this case illustrate informed choice?
2. How much detail and accuracy is the midwife required to provide to this potential client at a consultation?

3. When a client refuses a procedure or test that the midwife thinks is necessary, what should be done?
4. How should the midwife proceed from this point?

Analysis

This case illustrates the process of informed choice in that the woman and her midwife share in the responsibility of her care. The educated client is likely to take an active role in her birth plan. The depth with which a client becomes engaged in her care is reflective of the midwife-client relationship. To facilitate informed choice, a midwife offers informed consent and collaborates with the client in making decisions regarding every aspect of care. The client who exercises informed choice asks questions, researches issues pertaining to her care, and provides input to the midwife. Together, the midwife-client system works to make choices that are shared.

Informed choice begins at the initial contact of midwife and potential client. During the consultation or interview, the midwife has an ethical obligation to provide a client with accurate information to a depth of detail that protects the interests of both parties. A potential client may express a desire to work with a Christian midwife. The midwife may not be comfortable sharing her religious views, and is thus not required to do so. Yet, she is ethically bound to be honest in answering questions, and should not mislead the client. In Case 4, Melinda clearly desires a midwife of a specific style and expertise with water birth. The midwife should give an honest answer to her questions in regard to her comfort and experience with water birth and her style, even if she may lose the potential client by disclosing a conflict of style or comfort with the woman's preferences. Providing honest, accurate information respects the woman's right to informed choice and reflects the MMOC.

When a midwife is uncomfortable with a client's choices, she has a few options. First, she must communicate her discomfort to the client, along with the reasons for her disagreement and possible alternatives. Then, she should consider the ramifications of proceeding with the client's decisions. In case of refusal for a group B strep screen, both parties are protected by the existence of a signed informed consent document demonstrating the risks and benefits of the screening and the client's written refusal. If the midwife is comfortable with the client taking this risk, there is no need to change care.

Melinda's midwife did not object to not performing the group B strep screen, but she clearly objects to the client's unwillingness to have a vaginal exam during labor. In this situation, the midwife should communicate her discomfort and reasoning for the vaginal exam to Melinda. Alternatives to an exam should be explored, such as continuing to labor without an exam or going to the hospital for a sonogram, which will likely result in a transfer of care. If Melinda still refuses, the midwife should document the client's refusal—either through charting it or in a written statement from the client.

If the midwife feels that the baby is in danger and the client refuses a procedure or transfer that could save the baby, the midwife's hands are tied. In our local jurisdiction, midwives are trained to call an ambulance. The ethics of this are questionable, but it does serve to protect some of the parties in the dilemma: the midwife and the baby. It is advisable for midwives to prepare for this scenario at the onset of care through a written agreement for transport or transfer in case of emergency situations.

INFORMED CONSENT GUIDELINES FROM THE NORTH AMERICAN REGISTRY OF MIDWIVES

The North American Registry of Midwives (2008) has published a list of elements that should be included in informed consent documents. The following list is provided to assist in the development of an informed choice/consent document for your practice:

1. a description of the midwife's education and training in midwifery, continuing education, and Peer Review process;
2. the midwife's experience level in the field of midwifery;
3. the midwife's philosophy of practice;
4. antepartum, intrapartum and postpartum conditions requiring consultation, transfer of care and transport to a hospital (this would reflect the midwife's written practice guidelines) or availability of the midwife's written guidelines as a separate document, if desired and requested by the client;
5. a medical back-up or transfer plan;
6. the services provided to the client by the midwife;
7. the midwife's current legal status. *Completion of NARM Certification cannot be seen as legal protection because legality is determined by state or provincial law;*
8. explanation of treatments and procedures;
9. explanation of both the risks and expected benefits;
10. discussion of possible alternative procedures and treatments and their risks and benefits;
11. documentation of any initial refusal by the client of any procedure required by law and follow up teaching plan;
12. availability of a grievance process; and
13. client and midwife signatures and date of signing.

(NARM, 2008, p. 55)

REFERENCES

American College of Nurse-Midwives (ACNM). (2004). *Code of ethics*. Silver Spring, MD: Author.

Gottlieb, M. C. (1997). An ethics policy for family practice management. In D. T. Marsh & R. D. Magee (Eds.). *Ethical and legal issues in professional practice with families* (pp. 257–270). New York: Wiley.

International Confederation of Midwives (ICM). (2003). *Code of ethics*. Retrieved January 30, 2009, from http://www.internationalmidwives.org/Documentation/Coredocuments/tabid/322/Default.aspx

Kaufman, T. (2007). Evolution of the birth plan. *Journal of Perinatal Education: Advancing Normal Birth, 16*(3), 47–52.

Kirsch, I. S., Jungeblut, A., Jenkins, L., & Kolstad, A. (1993). *Adult literacy in America*. National Center for Education Statistics. Washington, DC: U.S. Department of Education.

Lasser, J., & Klose, L. M. (2007). School psychologists' ethical decision making: Implications from selected social psychological phenomena. *School Psychology Review, 36*(3), 484–500.

Lerner, J., & Keltner, D. (2000). Beyond valence: Toward a model of emotion-specific influences on judgment and choice. *Cognition and Emotion, 14*(4), 473–493.

Lützén, K. (1997). Nursing ethics into the next millennium: A context-sensitive approach for nursing ethics. *Nursing Ethics, 4*(3), 218–226.

Midwives Alliance of North America (MANA). (1997). *Statement of values and ethics*. Washington, DC: Author.

National Association of Certified Professional Midwives (NACPM). (2004). *Essential documents of the National Association of Professional Midwives*. Retrieved October 3, 2008, from http://nacpm.org/a-z-index.html

North American Registry of Midwives (NARM). (2008). *Candidate Information Bulletin*. Lilburn, GA: Author.

Pope, K. S., & Vasquez, M. J. T. (1991). *Ethics in psychotherapy and counseling*. San Francisco: Jossey-Bass.

Rothman, B. K. (1979). *Two models in maternity care: Defining and negotiating reality*. New York: New York University Press.

Smith, C. A., & Lazarus, R. S. (1993). Appraisal components, core relational themes and the emotions. *Cognition and Emotion, 7*(3/4), 233–269.

CHAPTER 5

Who Is the Client?

CLIENT DEFINITION AND RESPONSIBILITY

Who is the client? This may be the most basic and fundamental question that we ask, for the answer guides ethical practice in fundamental ways. Impulsively, we respond to the question by stating that the pregnant woman under our care is the client. Although this may be accurate, a deeper exploration suggests that this may be but a partial answer. As we will see in the following discussion, this question is deceptively simple. When we ask "Who is the client?" we're also asking another question that has serious implications for ethical decision making: *To whom is the midwife primarily responsible?*

The professional midwife knows and understands that there are many individuals who are, if not clients themselves, "client-like." A short list of people who could be considered clients or client-like includes, but is not limited to, the following:

- Mother
- Fetus/baby
- Partner/spouse
- Client's parents/in-laws
- Client's children
- Other significant individuals in the client's life

Depending on the nature of the relationship, the involvement of various constituents during pregnancy and birth, and the midwife's view of each person's role, the degree to which any individual is considered client-like will vary. However, the question remains critical for midwives working with so many people: What are my ethical responsibilities to each of these parties, and with whom do my ethical obligations primarily lie?

The question becomes even more complicated in settings in which other care providers are present, such as hospitals and birthing centers. Although a midwife working in a hospital would not think of a physician as a client, ethical responsibilities to other professionals in the workplace certainly exist. We are also aware of our relationship to employers and institutions and that these connections can pose ethical challenges. We address these potential problems in greater detail at the end of this chapter. For now, we focus on the question of defining the client and the implications of having primary responsibilities to a single client (or client unit).

Primary Responsibility to the Client

Once we define our client, we make a de facto statement that, given an ethical conflict or dilemma, *we affirm our commitment to our client first*. Although others may have interests at stake, the midwife's primary obligation is to her clients. For example, a midwife working within a group practice has a primary commitment to her clients over her partners. If a client files a complaint against a partner in the practice, the midwife has an ethical obligation to make decisions based on the client's needs and well-being rather than those of her partner. When the interest of a client conflicts with the interest of a professional colleague, institution, or even our own, the client trumps all. This is not to suggest that the client is always right in such disputes, but rather that our commitment to our clients is primary. The midwife is advised to keep professional and personal bias in check so that the client can be treated justly.

Perhaps the most challenging situation arises when a midwife's own interests conflict with those of her clients. Many practicing midwives have had to face the challenges of meeting clients' needs over those of her own and those of her family (Bourgeault, Luce, & MacDonald, 2006). When a labor call comes during a birthday party, holiday, or family challenge, the midwife is bound by her professional responsibility to leave all behind to serve the client and attend to her needs above those of others. Other situations arise in the context of care—for example, when a midwife's need to protect her professional standing in an institution or organization conflicts with her client's immediate needs in care, such as a midwife advocating for a client in labor who does not want an episiotomy despite the doctor's or hospital's protocols. As midwives, we agree that our clients' needs come first, even when they conflict with our own needs. However, a midwife has an obligation to herself and others that must be counterbalanced with this overarching principle. In a recent study of midwives' reasons for discharging clients, "obnoxious or abusive behavior to staff/provider" was one of the most prominent justifications reported for termination of care (Schorn, 2007, p. 470). When a midwife's sense of safety and well-being are impaired by a client's behavior, negotiations of priorities or discharge may be necessary. An abusive relationship that threatens the midwife's functioning, whether professional or personal, necessitates reprioritizing.

More subtle challenges to personal boundaries may require a midwife to reexamine her priorities. This may take place in a legal context, when an ethical obligation to a client challenges the midwife's legal status. One can imagine a situation in a homebirth practice in which a client's immediate postpartum hemorrhage necessitates the dispensation of a medication for which the midwife is not licensed to use. Although it is in the midwife's scope of practice, the law does not permit her to dispense it. A midwife who goes beyond legal boundaries may be at risk of losing her license, and her other clients may suffer as a result. No one particular client's needs should jeopardize those of other clients. That being said, there are always exceptions, and an urgent need of a particular client may override those that are not urgent. The midwife is constantly renegotiating needs and balancing her primary responsibility to clients. Chapter 6 includes more information regarding boundaries, and Chapter 9 discusses noncompliance and termination of care.

We also want to acknowledge that midwives have ethical obligations to nonclients that should be maintained whenever possible. That the midwife has primary ethical obligations to her clients does not mean that she can disregard her ethical obligations to others. We always aspire to meet all of our ethical obligations, but recognize that the realities of daily practice sometimes force us to make choices; when such situations arise, we put clients first.

Establishing a clearly defined client is essential for ethical practice. Failure to do so may result in misunderstanding, confusion, and harm. Such problems may be the consequence of assumptions made by midwives, mothers, and others about the nature of professional relationships and obligations. For example, suppose that a pregnant woman and her female partner assume that they are a client unit, but the midwife assumes that the pregnant woman's partner is ancillary and "not really the client." If these assumptions go unstated, the partner may feel excluded and even mistreated. Care should be taken to communicate openly about the nature and limits of our professional relationships to avoid misunderstanding and promote harmony.

Properly defining the client has far-reaching implications for ethical practice, because it ultimately affects several other critical ethical principles and guidelines. For example, we have an ethical obligation to maintain confidentiality with clients. We ask again, *Who is the client?* The answer to this question will help us identify the limits of our confidential relationship. By actively involving mothers in the process of determining who they consider to be part of their client system (e.g., partner, sister), we can clarify and negotiate the understanding of "client" and the practical implications of drawing lines.

THE MOTHER-BABY UNIT

In most helping professions, the client is defined as an individual. For example, the client in medicine is the patient. Similarly, a psychologist's client is typically an individual, although family systems therapy conceptualizes the family unit as the client. A review of ethical guidelines in midwifery suggests that many midwives view the mother-baby unit as the client. For example, the National Association of Certified Professional Midwives (NACPM) notes that its members "recognize the inseparable and interdependent nature of the mother-baby pair" (2004, p. 1; see Appendix E). Similarly, the Midwives Alliance of North American (MANA) reports in its Statement of Values and Ethics that "we value the oneness of the pregnant mother and her unborn child - an inseparable and interdependent whole" (1997, p. 1; see Appendix A). That such language is absent from the International Confederation of Midwives' Code of Ethics (2003; see Appendix D) suggests that the client as the mother-baby unit may be a cultural conceptualization. The notion of the mother-baby unit as the client provides a frame of reference for midwives that informs and sometimes complicates ethical practice.

The unique state of pregnancy presents ethical situations specific to maternity healthcare providers, given the phenomenon of the mother-baby unit as client. The well-being of both mother and fetus are of concern at all stages of maternity care. At times, these may conflict, such as in the case of an Rh-negative mother, whose physiology may reject a fetus through Rh sensitization if prophylactic Rho-gam was not administered properly. Rho-gam is a blood by-product that is not free of risk for the mother. The midwife does not make this decision, but informs her client of the risks and benefits to both her and her fetus or future fetuses. The weighing of maternal and fetal risks and benefits arises at other times in maternity care. In obstetric practice, the decision to have a cesarean section is often made for the benefit of the baby, but risks to the mother must also be considered. In very rare circumstances, this incongruity of needs reaches a point at which the fetus's well-being must be weighed against the mother's survival and the needs of her other children and family (Draper, 2004).

Considering the mother-baby unit as the client brings other noteworthy concerns to light. Serving a mother-baby unit requires us to think differently about our professional relationships and ethical obligations, given that the pregnant woman and her fetus are conceptualized as a system rather than two individuals. As a system, the whole is greater than the sum of its parts, and the individual components of the system have reciprocal influence on one another (Capra, 1996). In this regard, we should ask not only how a particular treatment might affect the mother or the baby, but also how it might affect the mother-baby unit.

In the case of prophylactic intrapartal antibiotics, the mother-baby unit is protected against certain foreign pathogens that may present a risk to either party, but the entire system is affected by the treatment. As a result of treating the system, mothers may have an allergic reaction to the medication. Another possible consequence is that mothers may develop a yeast infection, resulting in babies developing thrush, among other potential outcomes. Because the mother and baby are inextricably bound, the effects on one part of the system cause changes in the other. Such is the case when a baby who develops thrush passes it to the mother during breastfeeding. Similarly, if the mother has an allergic reaction to antibiotics, the fetus is likely to be affected. In an extreme case of maternal anaphylactic shock, fetal hypoxia may result. These examples demonstrate how the mother-baby unit informs maternity care.

During the postpartum period, midwives continue to view the mother and baby as a system. This is consistent with the Midwives Model of Care (MMOC) (Rothman, 1979), as opposed to the medical model or technocratic approach. Despite the birth event that separates the mother on one physical level from the baby, the unit is still salient. Whereas obstetricians and pediatricians have discrete roles as providers for the mother and baby, respectively, the midwife remains the sole care provider for the mother-baby unit in many practice settings. In a hospital, where the mother and baby separation typically occurs, nursery staff attend to the babies' needs, and decisions regarding neonatal care are routinely made without maternal input. Midwives understand the biosocial effects of separating a baby from his or her mother. Neonatal tachypnea is a prime example. Lactation consultants and midwives agree that skin-to-skin contact is an effective measure to alleviate this variation (Trotter, 2005). This physiological response in the newborn underscores the unitary nature of mother and child.

CULTURAL CONSIDERATIONS

Cultural and social factors shape the way we see and understand the world, and in turn affect our practice. For example, Thompson (2003) noted that "the being of persons as persons is possible only through how they see themselves and how others see them" (p. 590). By extension, the being of clients (or client units) is possible through negotiated and shared meaning-making by which midwives, mothers, and significant others stake out the boundaries of "client." This process often happens independent of our efforts, but may be enhanced through active participation. If the midwife always views the client as the mother-baby unit, she should communicate this conceptualization clearly so that there are no unstated assumptions.

We also recognize that not all clients necessarily share the view of the mother-baby unit as inseparable and interdependent. This may be due in part to cultural factors that influence the conceptualization and understanding of pregnancy, motherhood, and the status of the fetus or baby. Midwives should be sensitive to clients' worldviews and refrain from imposing their constructions of pregnancy on others. This cultural sensitivity is consistent with our general respect for autonomy. (See Chapter 10 for a more detailed discussion of diversity issues.)

In a hospital setting, where the medical culture dominates, midwives' training often conflicts with those of other healthcare professionals, creating cultural strain for those who interface between the medical and midwifery models. A medical view of pregnancy involves two discrete patients. The mother's health and well-being are frequently treated separately from those of her fetus. Midwives working in hospital settings often find themselves straddling two paradigms: the MMOC and the medical model. We acknowledge the challenge of having one foot in each of these different worlds. Rather than offering a solution to this situation, we encourage midwives to reflect on their perceived position and role. Ultimately, "midwives' interpretation of their role in childbirth will determine their ethical approach and relationship with others" (Thompson, 2003, p. 590).

THE ROLE OF THE MIDWIFE

Professional midwives may hold multiple roles, including direct care provider, childbirth educator, managerial staff at a hospital, midwifery or nurse educator, and administrator, among others. Maintaining multiple roles involves inherent conflict of roles. When roles conflict, the definition of client becomes murky. A midwife may simultaneously serve more than one client, or she may represent childbearing women in a broader community sense, such as a childbirth advocate.

Jones (2004) describes the conflict of roles that midwives face in terms of a conflict of duties. Duties of equal importance may be prioritized in relation to contextual factors (i.e., circumstances). For example, when a midwife switches from the role of a primary care provider to that of a labor delivery nurse or doula, her primary duty may still lie with the client, but her role in serving the client is mitigated by job descriptions and hierarchy. Further role conflict in solving moral dilemmas arises when one's sense of duty clashes with that which is practical. For instance, if a woman with an undiagnosed breech presentation refuses transport to the hospital in a state where breech home birth is illegal, a midwife may choose a practical (utilitarian) approach over a sense of duty (deontological). Rather than attempt the breech birth at home, she may call an ambulance and continue care until its arrival. This way she may avoid potential damage to her practice and to midwives in her community, sacrificing the service of one client (the mother with the breech baby). Although the general rule of "client first" exists, individual midwives must weigh the benefits of such an approach with the situational factors that arise in different roles and contexts.

How the midwife defines the client is, in part, determined by her role. This in turn affects her priorities and the care that she provides. Maintaining multiple roles has potential for role confusion. Midwives who work in contexts with other healthcare professionals are likely to experience role confusion. In a clinic setting with physicians, partners, nurses, and staff, a midwife's role may be defined more narrowly than in practices where midwives work independently. This may minimize confusion in relation to duties, but it may increase tension between roles that are defined by relationships. Relationships with business partners may clash with client relationships when a client dislikes or has a preference for one of the partners. A midwife in this situation has to prioritize the client relationship while working to preserve the partner relationship.

Similarly, when a midwife works with nurses in a labor and delivery unit, nurses may have more direct contact with the woman in labor. The midwife may experience role tension when a nurse makes decisions about a client's care without consulting the midwife. This relationship may be informed by whether she has direct supervision over nursing staff. The fewer structural definitions surrounding roles, the more potential there is for conflict. If the midwife is simultaneously overseeing the care of two or more laboring women, she may have to prioritize among them based on their stage of labor and other contextual factors, such as risk status; this may further inform her role in each woman's care, leaving nursing staff in charge in some situations while the midwife is attending to other clients.

In these settings, and in others where roles mitigate relationships, the midwife-client relationship may be challenged. Yet, when clarifications are made in the informed consent process, the client is better equipped to deal with role confusion. It behooves the midwife to communicate to the client about mitigating relationships so that the client is fully informed and can ask questions and make the appropriate psychological adjustments.

CASE EXAMPLES

CASE 1

Danny contacts a midwife for midwifery services and arranges a consultation for himself and his wife, Shelly. At the consultation, Shelly is quiet and defers to Danny frequently. At the onset of care, it is clear that Danny is very involved in the pregnancy. He attends all prenatal appointments. When a question regarding informed consent arises, Shelly defers to Danny. For example, the midwife asks Shelly if she would consent to a vaginal exam and Pap smear during pregnancy. She discusses the risks and benefits of the Pap smear, clarifying that it could be postponed until the postpartum period because Shelly has never had an abnormal Pap and her most recent Pap was a year ago. Shelly turns to Danny, who states, "It sounds like a good idea; let's go ahead and get the Pap." Shelly nods back to the midwife. Even though the midwife is uncomfortable with the situation, because she feels that her client is unable to truly consent if she defers to her spouse, she performs the Pap smear.

A few months later, the couple attends a childbirth class, and brings a birth plan to the midwife that includes several boundaries. Danny explains, "We don't want anybody coming in the room except the nurse on duty and you. We don't want anybody to touch her except you and the nurse." The midwife, who works in a practice with doctors and other midwives, explains that another care provider may attend the birth. It could even be someone that they have never met.

Danny is visibly upset by this information. He is concerned about his wife's comfort with strangers. He requests that the midwife agree to attend their birth regardless of the call schedule. The midwife does not agree to this. Danny appears angry, and Shelly begins to cry. Despite her explanations of the nature of her practice, the couple seems disappointed and leaves the appointment without scheduling another prenatal visit. The midwife does not hear from them again, despite several attempts to reach them.

Questions

1. What ethical considerations are relevant to this case?
2. How could the midwife have defined the midwife-client relationship more clearly?
3. Could the outcome have been different if the midwife-client relationship had been clearly established?

Analysis

Both informed choice and confidentiality are at stake in this scenario. The midwife was unsuccessful in getting consent from the client, to whom she is primarily responsible, largely because she was unable to speak directly to the client without interference from the spouse. She should not have performed the Pap smear until she was absolutely sure that Shelly consented. The best way to achieve this may involve asking the partner to step out of the room. In this case, Danny seems very dominant, and may not be willing to remove himself. If the midwife suspects abuse, she has an additional ethical responsibility to the client to determine whether this is the case and to refer her to the appropriate agency for assistance. A tangential informed consent issue arose over the lack of clarity about the midwife's availability for births. This may not have related directly to the issue of who is the client. When the client is not clearly defined, ethical dilemmas can be difficult to solve.

The midwife could have taken a more active role in defining the client by directly discussing the issue with the couple. When Danny began answering questions directed at Shelly, the midwife had an opportune moment to discuss the nature of the clinical relationship between the client and the midwife. She could have further delved into issues of consent, explaining to the couple that unless she were certain that Shelly herself consented, she could not ethically provide services. The couple at hand is presenting themselves to the midwife as a unit. The midwife must then consider whether she is comfortable with accepting both the husband and wife as a client unit. Because Danny seems to be the representative of the couple, the midwife may require further proof of Shelly's agreement with his words, or ask that she answer some questions directly. If a midwife decides to accept this client unit, she will need to communicate to both Shelly and Danny the importance of input from both parties in making decisions about care.

Discussing the nature of the clinical relationship is well worth the time and effort. It provides an opportunity for all parties to chime in with their input regarding client definitions. A midwife may begin such a conversation by stating, "Now that you've hired me, our relationship begins to change. I now have ethical obligations to you and your baby as my client. Often, the client relationship includes the other parent of the baby. Do you expect this to be the case in your care?" If the midwife in Case 1 had begun a similar conversation at the onset of care with Shelly and Danny, perhaps she would have gained more clarity regarding their relationship and joint expectations for care. She certainly would have been able to address her concerns about Shelly's deferral to Danny in the consultation. Because their termination of care seemed to be tied to the midwife's call rotation, it is unlikely that such revelations about the clinical relationship would have kept them in her care.

CASE 2

Victoria attends her first prenatal visit with her midwife at a birthing center when she is 20 weeks pregnant. While taking the client's history, the midwife discovers that Victoria has been smoking throughout the pregnancy. The midwife reviews the risks of cigarette smoking with Victoria, but she is not receptive to quitting. The midwife attempts to negotiate with Victoria by encouraging her to cut back her use from a pack to half a pack per day. Victoria makes no promises, but the midwife is hopeful that a change will occur by the next visit.

When Victoria returns for her monthly prenatal visit, the midwife inquires about changes in the mother's smoking habits. Victoria reveals that she made a half-hearted try to cut back, but insists that her baby is fine. She goes on to tell the midwife that her own mother had smoked during her pregnancies, and all of the children were healthy. The midwife listens to her client's justifications, but is dissatisfied with her behavior. Again, she reviews the risks of smoking with the mother. She relates her concerns for Victoria's baby, to whom she is also responsible. Victoria remains resistant to altering her smoking behavior.

Questions

1. How can this midwife proceed with clinical care for the mother-baby unit when the mother refuses to accept appropriate medical advice?
2. Is there a point at which the midwife's obligation to the fetus requires her to prioritize its need over the mother's?

Analysis

All midwives have experienced situations in which a mother behaves in a manner that does not support the well-being of the baby. Typically, these situations revolve around nutrition and lifestyle. When an addiction, such as a nicotine addiction, is present, the mother-baby unit is illuminated. The midwife has an obligation to care for both fetal and maternal health, yet she cannot make decisions for a client regarding lifestyle. The woman remains an independently functioning adult, and her rights as such remain regardless of her behavior. Further, the midwife cannot ethically deny the mother her rights as a client. She owes her client confidentiality and informed consent, among other ethical obligations. To fulfill her obligation to the mother-baby client, the midwife must ensure that the mother understands the risks of her addictive behavior for herself and her baby.

Some midwives refuse to work with women who smoke, and will require clients to quit in order to continue care. In this situation, the midwife must balance her own values and protocols with those of her clients. A midwife may choose to transfer a client to a more appropriate provider if a baby is at high risk for low birth weight related to maternal smoking. Yet, transfer of care is unlikely to solve the problem for the mother-baby unit. The mother will likely continue smoking. We deal further with the ethical implications of transfer of care in Chapter 9. Here, we consider our dilemma when maternal behavior is a serious encroachment on fetal development.

If Victoria had an addiction to a more teratogenic substance, such as alcohol, how should the needs of the developing fetus be weighed with those of the mother? The midwife's obligation to the mother does not change, but her priorities may. If a mother is clearly exposing her fetus to harmful substances, the midwife must consider intervention for the health of the developing baby and the function of the mother-baby unit. At a minimum, the healthcare professional should refer the client for immediate counseling, attendance at Alcoholics Anonymous meetings, or some other professional service. Alternatively, the midwife can consider transfer of care. Legal obligations may also play a role in a midwife's action, especially in the case of a teratogenic substance.

CASE 3

Yongxia is considering midwifery care and home birth. She contacts a midwife by phone and schedules an appointment for a consultation. To the midwife's surprise, Yongxia arrives at the consultation with her parents, grandmother, sister, niece, and spouse. Because the midwife does not have a waiting room, all parties are present for the consultation. The midwife discloses that she is not accustomed to having so many people in a consultation and is not sure how to proceed. Over the course of the meeting, family members explain that they had been present for each other's births and functioned as a cohesive, extended family unit. Their plan is to be present and supportive for Yongxia throughout her prenatal care and birth, just as they had for other pregnancies and births in the family.

Following the consultation, the midwife spends a good deal of time reflecting on the meeting and thinking about the implications of an extended family-unit client. She is curious about cultural factors and the impact they might have on this family.

Questions

1. How can the midwife define the client with such a large group of participants in her care?
2. What would the midwife do differently if a complication arose during this woman's care?
3. What cultural implications are involved in this case?

Analysis

The midwife will need to collaborate with Yongxia in defining the client. Although there are many client-like persons in this case, the pregnant woman is the one to whom she owes the greatest priority. Because her primary responsibility is to her, she should look to Yongxia for clarity regarding inclusion of her family in her care. The midwife can maintain cultural sensitivity while working within a clearly defined clinical relationship to best serve her client.

There are too many implications involved for a midwife to treat the entire family as a client unit. For example, conflicts regarding confidentiality may arise. Further, it would be too time and energy consuming for the midwife to try to attend to all of the family members' needs during this client's care.

The midwife will need to make clear statements to the other family members about the nature of the clinical relationship and her role. She will need to get consent from Yongxia before disclosing confidential information at a prenatal visit, and will need further directives from Yongxia about communication with family members on the phone, in her absence, and at the birth. If a complication were to arise during Yongxia's care, the midwife should consider the input that she received from the client regarding her family's access to information and decision-making capacities.

To avoid miscommunication and promote understanding of her client's needs, it is also important for the midwife to seek information about the client and her family in regard to cultural traditions and mores. This will help the midwife prepare for unforeseen challenges that may arise over the course of care, and promote a sense of shared interest in the relationships with the client and her family.

REFERENCES

Bourgeault, I. L., Luce, J., & MacDonald, M. (2006). The caring dilemma in midwifery: Balancing the needs of midwives and clients in a continuity of care model of practice. *Community, Work, and Family, 9*(4), 389–406.

Capra, F. (1996). *The web of life: A new scientific understanding of living systems.* New York: Anchor Books.

Draper, H. (2004). Ethics and consent in midwifery. In L. Frith & H. Draper (Eds.), *Ethics and midwifery* (pp. 19–39). London: Books for Midwives.

International Confederation of Midwives (ICM). (2003). *ICM international code of ethics for midwives.* Retrieved November 3, 2008, from http://www.internationalmidwives.org/Documentation/Coredocuments/tabid/322/Default.aspx

Jones, S. J. (2004). Ethics and the midwife. In C. Henderson & S. Macdonald (Eds.), *Mayes' midwifery: A textbook for midwives* (pp. 1133–1141). London: Bailliere Tindall.

Midwives Alliance of North America (MANA). (1997). *Statement of values and ethics.* Washington, DC: Author.

National Association of Certified Professional Midwives (NACPM). (2004). *Essential documents of the National Association of Certified Professional Midwives.* Retrieved October 3, 2008, from http://nacpm.org/a-z-index.html

Rothman, B. K. (1979). *Two models in maternity care: Defining and negotiating reality.* New York: New York University Press.

Schorn, M. N. (2007). Midwives' practices and beliefs about discharging clients from their practice. *Journal of Midwifery and Women's Health, 52*(5), 465–472.

Thompson, F. E. (2003). The practice setting: Site of ethical conflict for some mothers and midwives. *Nursing Ethics, 10*(6), 588–601.

Trotter, S. (2005). Skin to skin contact: Therapy or treatment? *RCM Midwives Journal, 8*(5), 202–203.

CHAPTER 6

Multiple Relationships

The midwife-client relationship is best defined as a clinical one. A woman hires a midwife for her maternity services and pays the midwife for said services, and the midwife provides the agreed-upon services. This relationship, for the most part, has clearly defined boundaries: midwifery is a professional role involving direct care to a client during pregnancy, birth, and the postpartum period. Yet the unique context of childbearing may present greater potential for multiple relationships and challenging clinical boundaries than other healthcare fields. The increased intimacy inherent in the Midwives Model of Care (MMOC) (Rothman, 1979) presents potential relational conflicts that may threaten objectivity and pose potential harm. By paying greater attention to the nature of relationships, midwives can enjoy productive and satisfying interactions while protecting the interests of all parties.

Consider a rural midwife who provides services to people within her community: neighbors, friends, family, fellow church members, and acquaintances. This midwife will be challenged to protect her clinical relationships and must think carefully about the nature of her relationships with others. How can she effectively serve her community, make a living for herself, and protect personal and professional boundaries?

Relationships present many challenges. Clinicians must define the boundaries between personal and professional relationships. They must protect the interests of their clients, maintain objectivity in clinical judgment, and uphold ethical standards. To complicate matters, relationships are not static; they are constantly evolving and shifting. Hence, relationships require continual evaluation.

This chapter addresses the issues that midwives face in their professional relationships, including, but not limited to, relationships with clients, students, and colleagues. As clinicians, midwives must be aware of the potential for conflict in multiple relationships and in practical decision making when these conflicts arise. Moreover, midwives must learn to set professional boundaries, as well as develop the knowledge and skills to enforce them.

Consider the following vignette: Clarissa provides midwifery care to a small suburban population. Many of her clients are established acquaintances prior to entering a clinical relationship with Clarissa. Some are neighbors and/or fellow church members. Clarissa becomes aware of an extramarital affair involving a client's husband, who is also a friend of a friend. Clarissa is concerned for her client and is fairly certain that she is unaware of her husband's infidelity. She struggles with her knowledge of the affair and her concern for the well-being of the expectant mother.

The focal point of Clarissa's conflict is relational. How can she separate her roles and obligations? She has access to information that presents potential harm to her clients and her relationship with them. She must look to professional ethics to decide whether and how to act in this situation. Like all midwives, Clarissa must examine her relationships to maintain objectivity, competence, and effectiveness as a professional midwife.

Here, we review *multiple relationships* (sometimes called *dual relationships;* we use the terms interchangeably), boundaries, and the nature of professional relationships. This chapter does not address brief incidental or accidental contacts outside the clinical relationship, because these are not considered to be multiple relationships. For example, if you encounter your client at a public park, this does not constitute a dual relationship. Multiple relationships involve having both a professional and an additional relationship in which potential role conflicts exist.

PROFESSIONAL RELATIONSHIPS

How is a midwife's relationship with her client different from a midwife's relationship with a friend? How is your relationship with your neighbor different from your relationship with your dentist? What are the implications of being friends with your real estate agent? All of these questions focus on the nature of professional and nonprofessional relationships. We focus our discussion on midwives' professional relationships and the ethical considerations regarding dual or multiple relationships. A multiple relationship exists "if the professional were to assume another role in another relationship with the client" (Sonne, 2006, n.p.). Gottlieb (1993) defines dual relationships as those in which the clinician is in two role categories. According to role theory in social psychology, "a role is defined as the collection of expectations that accompany a particular social position . . . Each of these roles carries its own expectations about appropriate behavior" (Diekman, 2007, n.p.). As one might expect, the expectations that we have of a professional midwife are different from the expectations we have of a professional musician.

Multiple relationships present potential for both risk and benefit. Hence, "it is a fiduciary obligation to be in touch with risk factors, to manage them and minimize them" (Younggren & Gottlieb, 2004, n.p.). Midwives work in a variety of settings involving the potential for forming multiple relationships. In a hospital or birth center, a midwife on call may find herself serving a laboring woman with whom she has a prior relationship. A midwife who teaches childbirth classes may encounter a friend or neighbor enrolled in her class. In homebirth practices, many midwives assist other midwives in their communities. An assisting midwife may be called to attend the birth of a woman she knows through her child's school. As community health providers, midwives have a high probability of having a dual relationship with clients.

Your professional role and function may shape how you think about and behave in respect to multiple relationships. We can look to role theory to explain potential problems with dual relationships when "expectations attached to one role call for behavior incompatible with another role" (Kitchener, 1988, n.p.). The potential for incompatibility of roles is related to the potential for conflict in a multiple relationship. An obvious role incompatibility would involve a midwife providing maternity care to her psychotherapist. In a therapeutic relationship, the psychotherapist is an authority figure with whom the client shares her most intimate fears and dysfunctions. In a midwifery relationship, the midwife must make objective authoritative assessments and collaborate with the client as an equal. This would be very difficult for a midwife to achieve with her psychotherapist. A midwife cannot effectively serve a woman for whom she is also a psychotherapy client because the role incompatibility is high, as is the potential for harm to both parties. On the other hand, if your child's school custodian hires you for midwifery services, there is less role incompatibility. The school employs her, and your nonprofessional relationship is limited as a parent at the school. There is less role incompatibility and less potential for harm in establishing a midwife-client relationship.

Midwives can look to other healthcare professions for guidelines in identifying and managing multiple relationships. Psychology in particular has been very sensitive to multiple relationships. The following is the portion of the American Psychological Association's (2003) ethics code that addresses multiple relationships.

> **APA Ethics Code, Ethical Standard 3.05: Multiple Relationships** (a) A multiple relationship occurs when a psychologist is in a professional role with a person and (1) at the same time is in another role with the same person, (2) at the same time is in a relationship with a person closely associated with or related to the person with whom the psychologist has the professional relationship, or (3) promises to enter into another relationship in the future with the person or a person closely associated with or related to the person. A psychologist refrains from entering into a multiple relationship if the multiple relationship could reasonably be expected to impair the psychologist's objectivity, competence, or effectiveness in performing his or her functions as a psychologist, or otherwise risks exploitation

or harm to the person with whom the professional relationship exists. Multiple relationships that would not reasonably be expected to cause impairment or risk exploitation or harm are not unethical.

The APA code's treatment of multiple relationships is noteworthy for a number of reasons. The code defines multiple relationships broadly (see the three categories above), identifies the potential for impaired objectivity or harm, and acknowledges that there may be some multiple relationships that are not necessarily unethical. However, the code does not offer much guidance to practitioners who are in need of a decision-making model to help determine whether entering a dual relationship would be appropriate.

A couple of models have been proposed in the psychological literature regarding ethical decision making in dual relationships. These may be helpful for midwives to consider prior to entering a dual relationship with a client. We provide case examples at the end of the chapter where the following models can be applied.

Younggren & Gottlieb (2004) propose a decision-making model in which the clinician engages in an assessment and analysis of the necessity of the nonclinical relationship, the potential for exploitation, who benefits from the relationship, the risks of damage to both the client and the clinical relationship, and the clinician's ability to maintain objectivity; document the decision-making process; and obtain informed consent from the client prior to entering a dual relationship. The model can help clinicians to objectively analyze risk factors of a multiple relationship in which there is the potential for role incompatibility and inform their decision to enter into such a relationship. Guidelines for obtaining informed consent and related documentation protect both parties in the relationship.

In an earlier article, Gottlieb (1993) argues that the consumer's perspective must be considered in the process of deciding to enter into a dual relationship. His model (Table 6-1) involves considering three dimensions prior to entering a dual relationship: power, the duration of the relationship, and the clarity of termination of the relationship. The greatest potential for harm arises when the existing relationship involves a "clear power differential with profound personal influence," long duration, and indefinite termination (Gottlieb, 1993, p. 44). The proposed second relationship should also be viewed in consideration of these factors, and the potential harm assessed. If a decision to enter a dual relationship seems appropriate, Gottlieb insists that further steps be taken to ensure low incompatibility between roles, including seeking collegiate consultation and obtaining informed consent from the client.

Gottlieb's (1993) model is very user friendly and accessible for most multiple-relationship scenarios. The model's flexibility allows the clinician to apply the grid in Table 6-1 to both the current and proposed relationship, whether the ini-

Table 6-1   Dimensions for Ethical Decision Making

Low Power	Midrange Power	High Power
Little or no personal relationship *or* Persons consider each other peers (may include elements of influence).	Clear power differential present but relationship is circumscribed.	Clear power differential with profound personal influence.
Brief Duration	**Intermediate Duration**	**Long Duration**
Single or few contacts over a short period of time.	Regular contact over a limited period of time.	Continuous or episodic contact over a long period of time.
Specific Termination	**Uncertain Termination**	**Indefinite Termination**
Relationship is limited by time externally imposed or by prior agreement of parties who are unlikely to see each other again.	Professional function is completed but further contact is not ruled out.	No agreement regarding when or if termination is to take place.

Source: Gottlieb, M. C. (1993). Avoiding exploitive dual relationships: A decision-making model. *Psychotherapy, 30*(1), 41–48. Reprinted with permission.

tial relationship is clinical or personal. However, some relationships that fall in the middle of the grid or have a balance of variables to the right and left of the grid require further analysis, along with collegiate consultation for an objective outlook. If a case gets to the informed consent stage, the client is likely to benefit from access to the model. In any case, both models require the clinician who knowingly enters a dual relationship to continually monitor for potential harm and act accordingly.

The midwife should assess the client's vulnerability, strengths, and social support before entering into a second relationship (Sonne, 2006). Clients who have psychological disorders or limited ability to recognize, understand, and negotiate boundaries may be at higher risk in multiple relationships. Those who have been victims of sexual abuse may be particularly vulnerable. Unfortunately, most midwives have not been trained to screen clients for psychological problems and may not be well prepared to recognize symptoms. Nevertheless, midwives should do their best to assess client vulnerability and proactively avoid involvement in multiple relationships that may cause harm. Clients with internal and social strengths may be less vulnerable to potential harm from multiple relationships. As stated previously, clients can participate in decision making through the informed consent process (see Chapter 4 for more on informed consent).

BOUNDARIES IN PROFESSIONAL RELATIONSHIPS

Midwives who are considering entering multiple relationships should also consider the impact of the practice setting on relationships. For example, the implications of a midwife-client relationship outside the professional relationship might be different for a midwife in private practice than they would be for a midwife in a birth center or hospital, and rural practice frequently involves multiple relationships that would be very hard to avoid. We also must consider the setting of the nonprofessional relationship and the potential for harm. For example, the midwife who employs a client to clean her home may be less likely to experience significant negative outcomes from the nonprofessional relationship than the midwife who employs a client to manage confidential files in her practice.

Aside from multiple relationships, other professional boundaries are salient in a midwife's relationship with clients. Possible sites for boundary issues in a midwifery clinical relationship include protocols, time, and money.

Many midwives in private practice struggle to maintain financial boundaries with clients. Yet in some settings, money defines the business nature of relationships (Gutheil & Gabbard, 1993). The same may also be true for midwifery. Moreover, the nature of the midwifery relationship blurs the roles of work, friendship, and family. Some midwives see their work in light of service. Such a perspective, although altruistic, may actually present more risks than benefits to the midwifery relationship, especially when a payment for services is expected. A different set of financial boundaries are involved when a midwife knowingly takes a pro-bono client into care, because no material exchange is expected in return for services rendered. Yet, when a midwife fails to enforce contractual financial obligations, she unintentionally undermines the nature of the clinical relationship, leaving clients confused about roles and expectations.

The length of midwifery appointments also communicates boundaries to the client. If you typically set aside an hour for appointments but continually allow a client's appointment to run late, you are allowing a boundary to be breached. The consequences for doing so may be miniscule or grand. One midwife had a client who came to expect longer appointments, and when another client arrived for an appointment after an hour, the client in session felt betrayed. This sense of betrayal can permeate other aspects of the relationship. Unless the midwife decides to charge additional fees for appointments that regularly run overtime, she is allowing her own personal time to be consumed by a client at the expense of time the midwife could be spending with her own family or on other business. The client may begin to expect her to make additional sacrifices during the time of the birth, postpartum period, or thereafter, leading to potential harm to the relationship. The client may begin to confuse the midwife's role in her life and become dependent upon her as a primary source of social support, even if that is not desired on the part of the midwife, who has many other women in her care.

Following practice protocols is an important way that midwives define and enforce clinical boundaries. The MMOC places women as individuals at the center of care, yet midwives must structure services with evidence-based protocols. When a client refuses a treatment that the midwife thinks is necessary, a potential for conflict arises. The midwife can honor both her protocols and her client's right to freedom of choice through signed refusal statements, referral, transfer of care, or mediation. If a midwife recommends a newborn screen or ultrasound and the client refuses, it is in the midwife's best interest to protect her professional boundaries and have the client sign a refusal form. This documents the midwife's consistency with her protocols and the client's refusal, and it communicates the midwife's personal boundaries to the client. Other situations may require a midwife to take greater action in defense of her boundaries. If a midwife attending an out-of-hospital birth determines a need to transport to the hospital and the client refuses, the midwife may need to initiate emergency services by calling for an ambulance. By upholding practice protocols, a midwife can protect her clients, herself, and her practice from potentially risky boundary violations. We further explore client noncompliance in Chapter 9.

Setting and enforcing boundaries are important skills that uphold professional standards and reflect respect for oneself and others. Boundaries are essential in multiple relationships. Midwives can look to colleagues and other healthcare professionals for relevant clinical boundaries and apply them in the practice of midwifery.

CASE EXAMPLES

CASE 1

Felipe is a midwife in a U.S. border town who is also a licensed physician in Mexico. Felipe has a large extended family living on both sides of the border.

Julieta is a Mexican national who works in the U.S. border town. She has received prenatal care from a Mexican obstetrician, but at 36 weeks, she begins looking for a midwife in the United States, because she plans to deliver her baby there. She schedules an appointment with Felipe for a consultation. In the meeting, they discover that they are related as distant cousins. Felipe shares his concerns with Julieta about taking a family member as a client. Julieta doesn't feel that the relationship poses much potential harm, because they are only distantly related and had not met until this encounter.

Questions

1. How should Felipe decide whether or not to take Julieta as a client?
2. Who bears the greatest potential for harm in this dual relationship?
3. How can Felipe minimize the risk for harm once the clinical relationship is established?

Analysis

Considering Younggren and Gottlieb's (2004) model, the necessity of the relationship is a primary concern, because unnecessary dual relationships involve unnecessary risk. If Felipe is the only midwife available in the border town, then he should consider whether the dual relationship is exploitive. In the case of Julieta, it is unlikely that being her midwife would be exploitive. If there is potential for exploitation, a midwife should not accept the client into his or her practice. Next, Felipe must consider whom the dual relationship benefits. Usually, both client and clinician benefit from a clinical relationship: the client gets services, and the midwife gets paid. In this case, the one who serves to benefit the most from the relationship is Julieta, who desires her child to be born in the U.S. border town. Further considerations regarding the risk of either the client or the clinical relationship being damaged by the dual relationship must be explored. In this case, there is little risk because the family relationship is distant and there is no history of personal contact. Felipe now must reflect on his objectivity in the matter. It behooves him to consult with another healthcare professional. Sometimes, the law must be consulted as well.

Once Felipe decides to accept Julieta as a client, he must document his decision-making process, and ensure that Julieta gives informed consent regarding the risks of the dual relationship. This conversation should include possible conflicts that could arise, including the presence of other family members at the birth, future contact within family settings, and challenges to professionalism when a family relationship knowingly exists.

This case demonstrates how the decision to enter a dual relationship should be considered prior to entering a clinical relationship. Using Younggren and Gottlieb's (2004) model, the case shows little risk of harm to the client or the clinical relationship. Perhaps the greatest risk lies with the midwife. If Julieta is dissatisfied with Felipe's services, she may complain to her family members. If this level of risk is acceptable to Felipe, then there is no ethical reason to deny this woman services. However, it is important that Felipe practice risk management in the clinical relationship by monitoring and minimizing the potential for harm in the dual relationship over the course of Julieta's care.

CASE 2

Suzanne is a certified nurse–midwife practicing in partnership with several midwives and doctors at a birth center attached to a community hospital. Her friend from high school, Perry, is in her first trimester of her second pregnancy when she contacts Suzanne to schedule an appointment. Suzanne, aware of possible complications in a dual relationship, hesitates to schedule the appointment. She asks Perry if she would rather seek another midwife's services in the practice. Perry insists that she prefers Suzanne, whom she trusts greatly. Suzanne agrees to meet with her for an initial consultation.

Questions

1. Is Gottlieb's (1993) or Younggren & Gottlieb's (2004) model more applicable to this scenario?
2. What input should the consumer have in making a decision to enter a dual relationship?
3. How does role incompatibility affect the decision to take on a dual relationship?

Analysis

The history of the relationship between this midwife and her potential client lends itself well to Gottlieb's (1993) model. Initially, the consumer should assess the current relationship on the dimensions of power, duration, and termination. Typically, peers don't have large power differentials. The duration of Suzanne and Perry's relationship is probably long, and the relationship is not likely to be terminated soon. Because two of the three dimensions fall on the right side of the chart, the potential for harm is high and a clinical relationship would be inappropriate.

However, if Perry considers the friendship to be of intermediate duration, then consideration of the potential clinical relationship along each continuum may provide further insight. This may be the case if Perry and Suzanne have only seen each other a few times since high school graduation. Then, the new relationship can be analyzed in the same manner.

The second step is to examine the contemplated relationship in relation to power, duration, and termination. There is a clear power difference in the clinical relationship, with the midwife having considerable influence. The duration of the relationship is intermediate, with regular contact over the childbearing year, after which the clinical relationship has a specific termination—the six-week postpartum checkup—unless the client seeks annual well-woman care.

If both the present relationship and the contemplated one fall near the middle of the grid, one can continue to the next step in the model. Both relationships should be examined for role incompatibility. If there is a high degree of role incompatibility, then the new relationship should not be established. If the incompatibility is low, consultation from a colleague is necessary before proceeding. Finally, the consumer must review the decision-making process and provide informed consent of the risks inherent in the dual relationship.

If Perry and Suzanne's relationship is limited to class reunions and a few other interactions, then there is less incompatibility than if the two frequently vacation together and have regular social interaction. Thus, role incompatibility may be the decisive factor in this case.

Midwifery care may be extended to friends, family, and neighbors. This has been the case at The Farm in Sunnyville, Tennessee (Gaskin, 1990), as it was in early American history (Ulrich, 1990). It is important for midwives who serve those with whom they share multiple relationships to weigh the potential risks and benefits with these clients and take protective measures when appropriate. Objectivity can be completely lost when one is intimately serving a family member or friend during the childbearing year. Therefore, when serving loved ones, consultation with colleagues is the most important measure one can employ. A midwife peer can balance one's intimacy with the client with objectivity, and inform the care that the client receives.

CASE 3

Cynthia is a homebirth midwife practicing in her hometown. Her good friend Michelle is pregnant with her third child. Cynthia had assisted at Michelle's last birth as a midwife apprentice. Now that Cynthia is certified, Michelle wants to hire her to be the midwife for this pregnancy. Cynthia is excited about the possibility of working with her friend, but also concerned about the risks related to multiple relationships. After discussing these in depth with Michelle, they agree to proceed with the clinical relationship, with Michelle treating Cynthia as if she were any other midwife and Cynthia treating Michelle as if she were any other client.

When Michelle is unable to pay Cynthia for her services in advance, they agree to a payment system that works for both parties. Cynthia would like to offer Michelle a discount, but their prior agreement to uphold a professional relationship stands.

When Cynthia notices that Michelle's diet is less than satisfactory, she offers nutritional counseling, as she would to other clients. Yet, when the two of them dine together, there is awkwardness regarding Michelle's tendency to eat high-sugar processed foods. Cynthia chooses to ignore this behavior, limiting her discussion of diet to prenatal appointments. Yet, she feels that she has to set a good example, and thus avoids tempting sweets when they are together.

It seems that as long as both parties adhere to the agreed-upon professionalism, their role conflict is low. Over the course of the pregnancy, things continue to go smoothly in their friendship and clinical relationship. There is much excitement about the approaching birth.

When Michelle goes into labor, Cynthia goes over to attend her as she would any other client. She usually calls her apprentices to go on births, but Michelle prefers to keep the birth intimate, and Cynthia agrees to allow Michelle's sister, Donna, to assist her. Donna has had a home birth and has been present at Michelle's other births.

The first stage of labor proceeds normally. When dilation is complete, Michelle has no urge to push. She takes a nap. Cynthia continues monitoring the baby, and Donna prepares some food downstairs. When Michelle awakes, she moves around the house and squats occasionally. The baby sounds great. Michelle eats some food and drinks plenty of water. Her vitals are stable. After another hour, she starts to feel pushy. She squats, and the baby's head becomes visible. After a few pushes, the head comes to a crown, where it lingers and slowly starts to emerge. The head doesn't quite deliver, and a turtle sign is seen. Cynthia starts to worry. She tells Donna to bring the resuscitation equipment. Donna starts to worry and ask Cynthia questions. Cynthia manages the shoulder dystocia on her own, ignoring Donna and shouting orders to Michelle. The baby requires some resuscitation, and transitions well with blow-by oxygen within two minutes of the birth.

Questions

1. What is the major risk to this multiple relationship?
2. Where did Cynthia go wrong in managing this case?
3. What else could Cynthia have done to protect her and her client?

Analysis

Because Cynthia and Michelle are good friends, there is much at risk. Both the personal friendship and the clinical relationship are at risk by virtue of a dual relationship. Strain on one relationship would certainly pose potential harm to the other, as well as to each person involved. A clinician has an obligation to prioritize the clinical relationship, even when it poses a threat to the personal relationship, Cynthia must act according to her midwifery standards when providing care to Michelle. Perhaps the greatest obstacle in doing this well is lack of objectivity.

Cynthia and Michelle agreed to initiate care with full knowledge of the risks involved. They made a verbal contract to honor the midwife-client relationship, and Cynthia tried to treat Michelle as she would any other client. Yet, Cynthia misled herself about her ability to act objectively. In spite of her protocols, or typical mode of care, Cynthia did not call another midwife to assist her on Michelle's birth. When a complication arose, the sister-in-law was unable to fill the assistant's role, and the outcome of the baby may have been jeopardized. By not sticking to her boundaries, Cynthia endangered her client.

A midwife who takes on a multiple relationship with a client should seek consultation and collaborative care with another professional. This should be done prior to the onset of care and during both antenatal and postpartum care. In the case of home birth, another midwife should be present. This may also be true in other birthing locations where an objective second opinion and competent assistance is not accessible. In short, Cynthia should have sought consultation and collaboration with another midwife during Michelle's care, and she should have had another midwife at the birth.

REFERENCES

American Psychological Association (APA). (2003). *Ethical principles of psychologists and code of conduct.* Retrieved April 13, 2009, from http://www.apa.org/ethics/code2002.html

Diekman, A. B. (2007). Roles and role theory. In R. F. Baumeister & K. D. Vohs (Eds.), *Encyclopedia of social psychology*. Retrieved April 17, 2009, from http://www.sage-ereference.com/socialpsychology/Article_n457.html

Gaskin, I. M. (1990). *Spiritual midwifery*. Summertown, TN: Book Publishing Company.

Gottlieb, M. C. (1993). Avoiding exploitive dual relationships: A decision-making model. *Psychotherapy, 30*(1), 41–48.

Gutheil, T. G., & Gabbard, G. O. (1993). The concept of boundaries in clinical practice: Theoretical and risk-management dimensions. *American Journal of Psychiatry, 150*(2), 188–196.

Kitchener, K. S. (1988). Dual role relationships: What makes them so problematic? *Journal of Counseling and Development, 67*(4), 217–221.

Rothman, B. K. (1979). *Two models in maternity care: Defining and negotiating reality*. New York: New York University Press.

Sonne, J. L. (2006). *Nonsexual multiple relationships: A practical decision-making model for clinicians*. Retrieved April 17, 2009, from http://www.division42.org/MembersArea/IPfiles/Fall06/reprints/multiple_relationships.php

Ulrich, L. T. (1990). *The life of Martha Ballard, based on her diary*, 1785–1812. New York: Vintage Books.

Younggren, J. N., & Gottlieb, M. C. (2004). Managing risk when contemplating multiple relationships. *Professional Psychology, 35*(3), 255–260.

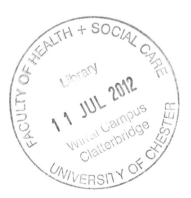

CHAPTER 7

Scope of Practice and Competence

SCOPE OF PRACTICE, COMPETENCY, AND THEIR LIMITS

As we continue our discussion of ethical decision making, we are continually reminded that professionals, clients, and observers do not always agree about the best or right course of action. After all, if the issues were clear-cut and easy to resolve, ethical codes and this book would be unnecessary. We acknowledge that many of the ethical standards in midwifery and other health-care professions lack controversy, debate, and opposition. Who is against confidentiality or informed consent? Rather, it is the application of these principles in the untidy world of daily practice that presents challenges, disagreements, and tough choices. Scope of practice and competency, the subjects of this chapter, are no exception.

Scope of practice and *competency* are used both in ethical and legal/regulatory contexts. From a legal/regulatory perspective, *scope of practice* is a limitation on the procedures and actions of a provider, usually determined by a licensing act or board. For example, in our home state of Texas,

> "Midwifery" means the practice of: (A) providing the necessary supervision, care, and advice to a woman during normal pregnancy, labor, and the postpartum period; (B) conducting a normal delivery of a child; and (C) providing normal newborn care. "Newborn" means an infant from birth through the first six weeks of life. (Texas Midwifery Board, 2005)

Such regulation is intended to limit the actions of a profession in the interest of ensuring that practitioners are properly trained, qualified, and licensed to provide services. Without scope of practice limitations, psychologists would be allowed to conduct a normal delivery of a child and midwives would be able to administer psychological tests. Thus, the limits on scope of practice are intended to keep professionals from practicing outside their professional duties.

Competency is a related but distinct issue and refers to a sufficient level of knowledge and skill to practice effectively. Training, both in didactic instruction and in the field, is designed to develop competency in the student of midwifery. For the established professional, continuing education keeps midwives' competency current with advances in the field. In this chapter, we explore both scope of practice and competency as important ethical issues. Most healthcare professionals are ethically bound to limit their practice to activities within their competency. For example, a midwife whose client presents with a mental illness should recognize that the diagnosis and treatment of the illness is outside her competency and make a referral to someone qualified in the diagnosis and treatment of such a problem. Here we present these issues in the framework of ethical practice.

Like other care providers, a midwife has an ethical responsibility to examine her competency to perform her role and function. Moreover, she must assess her competency to use an intervention, skill, or technique that is new to her (this concept has been applied to psychologists in Jacob and Hartshorne, 2003). In Chapter 10 we introduce the concept of *cultural competence*, or one's readiness to competently serve diverse populations. Ultimately, accurate self-assessment allows the midwife to determine not only her strengths but also her limits. As we mentioned in Chapter 1, "do no harm" is a cornerstone of biomedical ethics, and practicing beyond the boundaries of one's competency can result in significant harm.

When one considers the potential problems that could result from misdiagnosis or inappropriate intervention, the paramount importance of recognizing and respecting the boundaries of competency becomes obvious. When a boundary of competency is recognized, the ethical midwife seeks consultation and assistance from a midwife who has competency in the area of concern or refers the client to a provider who possesses the needed competence.

WHY EMPHASIZE SCOPE OF PRACTICE AND COMPETENCY?

The professional literature in midwifery addresses issues of competency and scope of practice repeatedly. The American College of Nurse-Midwives (ACNM) has addressed the issue in a position statement declaring that "Certified Nurse-Midwives (CNMs) and Certified Midwives (CMs) are providers of primary health care for women and newborns" (ACNM, 1997, p. 1). The document goes on to list "preconception counseling, care during pregnancy and childbirth, provision of gynecological and contraceptive services and care of the peri- and post-menopausal woman" as activities that fall under the care of CNMs and CMs (p. 1).

At first glance, the ACNM (1997) position statement appears to be directed at consumers and other care providers who may be unfamiliar with midwifery, as if to say, "This is what a midwife is and what a midwife does, in case you didn't know." However, placed in the context of similar documents and statements, the position statement seems to have other significant functions. This is particularly apparent in the Essential Documents of the National Association of Certified Professional Midwives (NACPM, 2004; see Appendix E). Although published documents are a source of public information, their primary function is to regulate midwives. Generated by midwives, ACNM's and NACPM's papers define the scope of practice for midwives as a means of self-regulation.

McCool and McCartney (2007) note that ACNM frequently receives questions about the scope of practice of a midwife. ACNM has published two additional documents that directly address competency and scope of practice: Core Competencies for Basic Midwifery Practice (ACNM, 2007) and Standards for the Practice of Midwifery (ACNM, 2003). These documents serve a critical function because they define competencies, scope, and standards of practice for midwives, the general public, and other professionals. However, the documents alone cannot fully address issues related to competency and scope of practice in the profession. Midwives play a crucial role as well.

A licensed or credentialed midwife has established at least a satisfactory level of competency to practice, but this does not mean that the boundaries of her competency will not be tested (in fact, we believe that *all* midwives have limits). Therefore, we differentiate between the published standards or competencies and the application of those standards or competencies to daily practice. McCool and McCartney (2007) go on to say that "it is vital to midwives offering safe and beneficial care that the time is taken to define one's scope of practice and then to actually practice accordingly" (p. 188). In this respect, each midwife has her own individual scope of practice. Educating midwives about this principle and including it in peer review can bring the practitioner in alignment with her scope of practice and competency.

Under the heading "Scope of Practice," NACPM notes that its members "offer expert care, education, counseling and support to women and their families throughout the caregiving partnership, including pregnancy, birth and the postpartum period" (NACPM, 2004, p. 2). This is consistent with ACNM's position statement, but with an added component: "NACPM members are trained to recognize abnormal or dangerous conditions needing expert help outside their scope" (p. 2). Here midwives are not only defined by what they do, but also by what they do not do: independently treat conditions outside their areas of expertise. The significance of this limit cannot be overstated, for it acknowledges that professionals have limitations.

The overlap of scope of practice and competency with other domains of ethics is noteworthy. For example, the College of Midwives of British Columbia's Code of Ethics (1996) states that "midwives shall inform their clients of the scope and limitations of midwifery practice" (p. 2). This element demonstrates the intersection between scope of practice and informed consent. Interestingly, the code addresses the limitations of midwifery *practice* rather than the limitations of the *practitioner.* We assume that midwives are a diverse group with considerable variation in knowledge, skills, and experience. Consequently, any given midwife will have her own scope of practice, defined in part by her training and experience, but also by her own unique limitations (ACNM, 2008). This is not to suggest that a midwife can unilaterally determine that her scope of practice exceeds that of her profession; rather, her own scope of practice falls within the profession's scope.

According to McCool and McCartney (2007), several other factors affect midwifery's scope of practice: state laws and regulations, federal agencies, third-party payers, healthcare facilities, litigation, and the midwife's "philosophy, ethics, experiences, and personality" (p. 188). Therefore, one would expect the scope of practice in midwifery to vary by state, facility, individual midwife, and so on.

Competency and scope of practice as ethical issues in midwifery should be conceptualized in terms of "*nonmaleficence* (a norm of avoiding the causation of harm)" and "*beneficence* (a group of norms pertaining to relieving, lessening, or preventing harm and providing benefits and balancing benefits against risks and costs" (Beauchamp & Childress, 2009, pp. 12–13). We prevent and avoid harm by recognizing our limits and making a commitment to stay within those limits. This relationship between recognizing and respecting the limits of competency and preventing or avoiding harm also relates to the idea of responsible caring, as discussed in Chapter 3 of this text (Jacob & Hartshorne, 2003).

In summary, defining scope of practice and competency serves multiple purposes. In drawing lines around the activities of midwifery and those activities that are beyond the scope of midwifery, the profession communicates the role of the midwife, establishes training goals and standards, sets expectations for consumers and other providers, and acknowledges that there are limits on what midwives can and should do. Next, we deal directly with issues related to competency.

DETERMINING AND MAINTAINING COMPETENCY IN MIDWIFERY

The ACNM Code of Ethics states that "to respect their own self-worth and dignity, midwives must understand the value and the limits of their own knowledge, beliefs, and emotions in professional interactions (ACNM, 2008, p. 4; see Appendix C). It is striking that ACNM sees competency in the context of self-worth and dignity. Clearly understanding one's limitations will undoubtedly serve clients as well, for a midwife who uses procedures beyond her skill set may have higher negative outcomes. Thus, the need to accurately assess one's competency and respect those limits is paramount.

The midwifery student's competency is continually assessed through course-work (tests and quizzes) and supervised fieldwork (apprenticeships, internships, etc.). A student seeking to become a midwife is required to pass licensing and certification exams to ensure competency before engaging in independent prac-tice. Once licensed or certified, midwives are still responsible for maintaining competency through required continuing education.

The ACNM Code of Ethics requires midwives to "maintain the necessary knowledge, skills and behaviors needed for competence" (2008, p. 11). Experi-enced professionals need to update their knowledge and skills regularly because the field of midwifery is constantly changing. Also in flux are other healthcare fields, society, and culture. Within the field of midwifery, standards of compe-tency as articulated by professional organizations change over time as well (ACNM, 2008).

Midwives continually self-assess their competencies and work with others to build and maintain knowledge and skills. Activities such as participation in con-tinuing education, conferences, and peer review enable midwives to keep abreast of current trends in the field, collaborate with other professionals, share infor-mation, and in turn become better midwives. Midwives should take time to re-view not only their own client data but also aggregate data published in research journals to learn from real cases. The American Nurses Association's Code of Ethics for Nurses (2005) conceptualizes competency building as "lifelong learn-ing" that encompasses "continuing education, networking with professional col-leagues, self-study, professional reading, certification, and seeking advanced degrees" (n.p.). This makes sense, given the ever-changing competencies in mid-wifery (Ament, 2007).

An additional component of competency that is not widely addressed in the midwifery literature is the relationship between responsibility and competency. According to the Nursing and Midwifery Council's Code of Professional Con-duct (2002), as a midwife "you must acknowledge the limits of your professional competence and only undertake practice and accept responsibilities for those activities in which you are competent" (p. 678; see Appendix F). Although the thrust of this standard is to engage in activities that fall within your competence, embedded in the statement is the idea of responsibility or accountability. Put an-other way, midwives engaging in activities within their scope of practice and competency must take responsibility for their actions.

Some midwives work in small communities and have very limited, if any, op-portunities for consultation and referral. This presents a significant challenge when the boundaries of competency are tested. Although it is certainly better to serve a client to the best of your ability than to abandon her in the interest of re-specting the limits of one's competency, other creative alternatives should be considered. Phone consultations with more experienced midwives who are not close enough for a face-to-face visit may assist a new midwife with emerging skills and competency. Similarly, the sharing of digital images across the Internet may assist in long-distance consultations regarding diagnosis and treatment. A word of caution: midwives must safeguard client privacy and confidentiality when communicating with others (see Chapter 3). Today's midwives have far greater options for consultation across vast distances than their predecessors.

PEER REVIEW

Like other ethical behavior, participation in peer review promotes professional autonomy for midwives. ACNM, the Midwives Association of North America (MANA), NACPM, and the International Confederation of Midwives (ICM) all uphold peer review as an ethical and practice standard. Peer review is an essential process for midwives to reflect on competency and scope of practice.

Rooks (2007) places the importance of peer review in the arena of self-regulation, upholding the philosophical belief, attributed to Aristotle, that a man should be judged by his peers. She describes the harsh disciplinary actions that commonly occur when the board of nursing regulates certified nurse–midwives. Instead, she advocates for peer review as the primary process by which midwives are held to competency standards. "Peer review is done for the purposes of quality assurance and improvement, not for fault finding or punishment; it does not focus on negative events or outlier values. Peer review is the professional responsibility of all midwives" (Ament & Tillett, 2007, p. 257).

The North American Registry of Midwives (NARM) published "NARM Community Peer Review: Community Peer Review Process," a guideline for Certified Professional Midwives (CPMs) in holding regular peer reviews (NARM, 2006). NARM regards peer review as the primary process by which midwives are held accountable for their behavior. Formal complaints should be addressed at peer review initially. NARM recognizes additional roles of peer review: validating the certification process, projecting an image of professionalism to the public, building community cohesiveness, and working toward proactive problem solving. NARM recommends decisions made by consensus, quarterly community peer review, inclusion of students, confidentiality, a supportive and educational atmosphere, and professional educational objectives for recertification. These guidelines demonstrate the importance of peer review to NARM, the certification body for CPMs. It is the responsibility of CPMs to uphold peer review standards in their communities.

In ACNM's (2005) position statement addressing quality management in midwifery care, peer review is defined as "the assessment and evaluation of midwifery practice by other midwives to measure compliance with ACNM standards" (p. 1). ACNM has developed an instrument for local chapters to use for peer review. Reviewers may do site visits, random chart review, and review of cases with poor outcomes (Ament & Tillett, 2007).

Although the purpose of peer review is professional self-regulation, improved professional knowledge and skills are a by-product (ACNM, 2005). This sentiment is echoed by Davis (2004): "Exposure to the standards and practices of others motivates participants to continually upgrade their knowledge and skill" (p. 247). Peer review promotes competency.

Professional organizations agree that peer review is a valuable tool for midwives. "Midwifery practice includes an on-going process of case review with peers" (MANA, 2005, p. 2). The NACPM member "informs each woman she serves of mechanisms for complaints and review, including the NARM peer review and grievance process" and "participates in continuing midwifery education and peer review" (NACPM, 2004, p. 4). ACNM's code of ethics "provides a framework for peer consultation and review and orients midwifery students to the moral obligations of the profession into which they are being socialized" (2008, p. 2). ICM (2003) states that "midwives develop and share midwifery knowledge through a variety of processes, such as peer review and research" (p. 2).

Ultimately, responsibility for competency and scope of practice rests with the midwife. Although training programs, professional organizations, and regulatory bodies establish practice guidelines and competencies, each midwife has an ethical obligation to know and respect her limits, not only for optimal client care but also for her own self-worth and the promotion of confidence in the profession.

CASE EXAMPLES

CASE 1

Nadine is a midwife practicing in a rural setting. She has been certified for three years, and she has occasionally worked with other midwives in her state, although there isn't another practicing midwife within 100 miles of her practice.

She has a client, Jenny, whose baby has been in a breech presentation since 32 weeks. As the time of the birth approaches and many of the corrective measures for breech presentation have been employed without success, Nadine considers external version. She is aware of the risks associated with external version and breech delivery, but she has not informed her client of these.

When Jenny comes in for her 36-week prenatal exam, the baby is still breech. Nadine begins to counsel Jenny about her options, including attempted external version, collaboration with a physician, breech delivery out of the hospital, and transfer of care to an obstetrician. She further informs Jenny that her chances of having a vaginal birth in the hospital are slim, should the baby remain in a breech presentation. Nadine admits that she has never attempted an external version, and that she has never witnessed a breech birth, although she is trained in breech delivery.

The client adamantly wants to avoid a hospital delivery, believes that breech births are normal, but wants to try to alter the presentation with external version in Nadine's office. She further explains that she trusts Nadine and wants her to deliver the baby out of the hospital, even if the presentation remains breech. She is a highly educated woman, whose partner is completely supportive, and Nadine thinks that she would be a good candidate for breech birth out of the hospital.

Nadine calls an experienced midwife in the state, who agrees to attend the breech delivery, but is unwilling to drive to Nadine's office for the attempted version. Nadine is able to convince her client to drive with her to the other midwife's office, over 100 miles away, to attempt the version there.

At that appointment, external version is unsuccessful. A second appointment is set to attempt the version the following week, and plans are discussed regarding the possible breech home birth. The experienced midwife reviews the risks and benefits of both breech birth and transferring care to an obstetrician. Jenny does not waver. She and her partner maintain that they desire an out-of-hospital birth. Nadine emphasizes the possibility that the other midwife may miss the birth, due to travel distance, and that she may be the only midwife at the birth. She asks the couple to sign a document outlining all of the risk factors discussed, and a refusal to transfer care to a physician. The couple does so willingly, and plans are made to continue attempts to turn the baby.

Questions

1. Why is breech birth such a controversial topic in the medical community in regard to scope of practice and competency?
2. Are there other areas of midwifery practice that bear the same level of scrutiny from the medical community in relation to scope of practice?
3. By utilizing informed choice, did the midwife "cover her bases" in terms of ethical conduct?
4. What is the role of the second midwife in this case study?
5. What ethical responsibilities does the second midwife have to the client and to her colleague, Nadine?

Analysis

Breech birth is a topic of much controversy in the birth community. Most obstetricians routinely deliver breech babies through planned cesarean section, avoiding the possibility of breech vaginal birth. As a result, many midwives feel that the only chance a woman has of a vaginal birth with a breech presentation is to have an out-of-hospital birth; thus, many midwives offer this as an option to their clients under specified conditions.

In this context, the midwife in our case example offers her clients a full range of choices, informing them to the best of her abilities about the risks associated with breech delivery. She admits her lack of experience with breeches and external version, initiating collaborative care with a more highly trained midwife. By emphasizing the possibility of her delivering a breech baby for the first time unassisted by another midwife, she further informs her client of risk. The midwife has the expectant couple sign an informed choice document outlining all risk factors, thus placing responsibility for the choice into the hands of the parents of the baby. In terms of informed consent, Nadine has covered her bases with this client. However, informed choice must be weighed with other ethical considerations in applied ethics, such as scope of practice and competency.

With her scope of practice limited only by laws governing her practice, Nadine chooses to focus her discussion with the parents on her own competency, as well as that of the other midwife. We do not specify the legality of breech delivery at home in this case study, because it varies from state to state. Some midwives work on another principle, *standard of care*, when making decisions regarding a controversial procedure, such as breech delivery at home, when laws are nonexistent, unclear, or unjust. Nadine rightly focuses the discussion on her lack of competency in both external version and breech delivery. By collaborating with another midwife, Nadine acknowledges that her knowledge and skills are insufficient for the route her clients have decided to take in this matter. However, the clients and the outcome of their decision are still Nadine's responsibility, unless she transfers care to the other midwife and resigns herself to an assistant role at the birth.

By not resigning her role as the primary midwife and agreeing to attend the birth, even if the other midwife is unable to attend, Nadine is knowingly agreeing to work outside her competency. Even though she was trained in breech delivery through models, simulations, lecture, and self-study, she has not acquired competency experientially. Working outside her area of competency places her clients at greater risk. If a bad outcome were to happen, the midwife may be scrutinized, and ultimately blamed, for knowingly assisting a breech birth with no previous experience in breech delivery. When midwives work outside their areas of competency, they jeopardize their professional standing and the field of midwifery. Still, many midwives justify such behavior to preserve the woman's right to vaginal delivery and out-of-hospital birth. Some hotbeds of controversy in midwifery practice are scope of practice issues that midwives and doctors struggle to preserve or limit (respectively). From this position, Nadine is taking a professional and personal risk to preserve the area of competency and scope of practice for midwifery.

CASE 2

Farah is a certified nurse–midwife in a group practice that serves a socioeconomically diverse population in a major metropolitan city. The midwives in her practice attend births at a birth center located within the county hospital. Many of the women she serves are recipients of Medicaid. Few have an existing relationship with a physician or other healthcare provider.

Over her years of practice, Farah has encountered many mental health issues among her patients. Most commonly, Farah observes cases of postpartum depression. On occasion, Farah has a patient with an existing condition, such as depression or anxiety. Typically, these patients have a mental health practitioner who provides therapy.

Farah has recently come to suspect an undiagnosed case of depression in a patient who is married with three young children. Delores is Mexican American, 28 years old, and living in poverty in a small urban project. She relies on public transportation to get to appointments, and is often late. She misses two appointments in a row before Farah decides to call her. When Delores explains that she hasn't been feeling well, Farah encourages her to come into the office immediately for an exam.

Farah reviews Delores's chart before she comes in, and notes a history of sexual abuse, unemployment, and a lack of formal education. When she sees Delores, she asks her about her well-being, her moods, and her diet. Delores reports that she has a hard time getting out of bed and doing housework. Her recent diet has been limited to canned and processed foods. Farah asks about the children, who are with a grandmother during the appointment, and Delores seems uninterested in discussing them. Throughout her exam, Delores avoids eye contact and responds to questions and comments with silence and nods. Farah gets very direct in her questioning, and asks Delores if she has been depressed. Delores responds in the affirmative, but offers no further explanation. Farah encourages her to take some time away from the children, go on regular walks, spend time with her husband, and improve her diet. In her midwifery notes, Farah charts as follows: Patient presented with mild depression; advised appropriately per diet, exercise and social support; will follow up as needed.

Questions

1. How are Farah's scope of practice and competency defined in relation to mental illness?
2. What are the competency and scope of practice boundaries of midwifery counseling?
3. At what point should a practitioner refer care of a patient with mental illness?
4. Is it appropriate to terminate care in certain cases?

Analysis

Depression is the "common cold" of mental illness, and thus most midwives will encounter it during their practice with some regularity. Many patients will present with a history of depression, and the midwife should screen these patients regularly for signs and symptoms of depression, such as feelings of hopelessness and worthlessness, loss of interest in activities that once brought pleasure, and hypersomnia (American Psychiatric Association, 2000). Although many midwives have taken at least one introduction course in psychology, few midwives are equipped to diagnose and treat depression.

If a midwife has a license to practice psychotherapy, she is uniquely qualified in mental health. Midwifery training alone does not, in any way, qualify a midwife to practice in the field of mental health. The scope of midwifery is limited to healthy pregnancy. A mental illness may present as much risk to a pregnancy as a serious medical condition, such as essential hypertension. It is not the midwife's job to diagnose or treat mental illness. If mental illness is suspected, the midwife has a responsibility to refer the patient to an appropriate mental health practitioner.

Midwifery counseling is limited to adjustment issues related to pregnancy, childbirth, and the postpartum period. Many women start their pregnancy with such issues. A woman with an unplanned pregnancy may have struggles communicating her condition to family members and seeking support from her community. Her midwife may be able to link her to resources that assist her adjustment, including books and support groups. Similarly, midwifery counseling may be an effective tool in providing social support and guidance to a mother who is adjusting to motherhood and breastfeeding. Midwifery counseling is one of the most important forms of support that a woman will have in her childbearing year, but it does not substitute for a mental health practitioner.

Midwives who work in a high-density city are likely to encounter mental illness frequently. It can sometimes be difficult to discriminate mental illness from the challenges associated with poverty and discrimination. In fact, many social factors, including poverty, increase the prevalence of mental illness. The rate of mental illness among some populations can be alarming. Yet, no practice or population is free of mental illness, and certainly depression crosses all social, ethnic, and economic barriers.

Because of the prevalence of mental illness, midwives should have some mental health training and a protocol for referring patients with suspected mental illness to a qualified mental health practitioner. The sooner the referral is made, the better, in terms of patient outcomes. Midwives should follow up with patients who were referred for mental illness, to ensure that an evaluation occurs. Whenever possible, midwives should establish collaborative care with mental health professionals. This relationship may improve patient outcomes and provide smooth referrals. Seeking a relationship with a therapist who has experience working with women in the childbearing year is preferable because his or her competency with the population is established.

If a client refuses mental health counseling despite repeated attempts by the midwife to refer the client, a transfer of care may be appropriate. Some women with mental health issues may be poor candidates for natural birth. Further, they may present a danger to themselves or others if they remain untreated. Concerns over abandonment may factor into the midwife's decision to transfer care of a client whose mental health is challenged. Caution must be taken, because a transfer of care can simply mean passing a challenging case onto a new practitioner who may be less knowledgeable about the client's needs. Such a transfer may be of no benefit to the client. If a midwife decides that a client's mental health needs are outside her competency, and collaborative care is not possible, it may be best to transfer the client to a more qualified practitioner who works in a setting better matched to the woman's safety and needs.

CASE 3

Terry works in a small private practice adjacent to a major medical center where she has hospital privileges. In routine lab work, she finds a 35-year-old primigravida client to have an elevated white blood cell count (WBC). At the next prenatal appointment, Terry discusses the labs with her client, Vanessa, who is in her 14th week of pregnancy and has no current signs or symptoms of illness or allergies. Terry follows up with a second complete blood cell count (CBC), where she finds the WBC values higher than before, with no other out-of-range values in the CBC. Although some rise in leukocytes is normal for pregnancy, the levels that she observes are inconsistent with normal trends.

Terry utilizes the resources that are available to her to interpret the lab work, but she is unable to find an adequate explanation for Vanessa's rising WBC. She consults with a midwife colleague, who suggests a round of antibiotics because an infection is likely. Terry also considers natural remedies to support the woman's immune system and fight infection, including increased vitamin C, probiotics, and herbal therapies.

Terry decides on a course of action that includes natural healing modalities followed by another CBC. When the WBC is even higher than before, she opts for broad-spectrum antibiotics, but this does not seem to significantly reduce Vanessa's WBC. Finally, Terry decides that because Vanessa is asymptomatic, no further course of action is necessary. She plans to run another CBC postpartum.

Questions

1. When abnormal labs are inexplicable, what should a midwife do?
2. With whom, if anyone, should a midwife consult or collaborate in this situation?
3. How do scope of practice and competency relate to interpretation of lab results and related treatments?

Analysis

Competency in laboratory testing and interpretation varies greatly among midwives. Some midwives apply greater focus on lab work than others, and they are likely to have more opportunities to develop related knowledge and skills. Consultation with an experienced colleague or referring physician can often aid interpretation of unusual lab results. Courses in basic lab interpretation are required for most midwifery programs, and sanctioned midwifery practice typically involves standard obstetric screens and tests. Thus, routine laboratory testing is within the scope of practice and competency of most midwives.

When a midwife reaches her limits of competency, she is ethically bound to consult, collaborate, refer, or transfer care. Consultation is often adequate when a midwife needs an outside or experienced opinion. Issues of confidentiality may be raised in the process. We explore the constraints of consultation and collaboration of care in Chapter 8. In this case scenario, Terry realizes that she is unable to process the lab findings and rightly consults with a colleague. Yet, because this colleague has not seen the client, and access to the chart may be limited, the advice that she gives is general, reflecting the consulting midwife's style of practice.

If consultation fails to effectively solve the problem, referral or collaboration may be required. The client's care should not be limited to the knowledge of her midwife. A midwife has a community of healthcare providers with whom she can work to meet a client's needs. In a case involving troubling lab results, referral to a physician makes sense. When consultation with the other midwife proved to be ineffective, Terry should have considered physician consultation or referral. The International Code of Ethics for Midwives states, "Midwives work with other health professionals, consulting and referring as necessary when the woman's need for care exceeds the competencies of the midwife" (ICM, 2003, p. 2; see Appendix D). Interpretation of lab work is no exception to this rule.

The midwife in this case scenario implemented treatment for her client without a diagnosis or adequate interpretation of lab work. Supporting the immune system with herbs and vitamins may be appropriate if infection is suspected, but antibiotic therapy is not without risk. If the mother develops subsequent infections due to invasive antibiotic therapy that was unnecessary, the midwife may actually cause harm to her client, including possible urinary tract infection and related risks. Ethical concerns arise over the responsibility of care for a client by a consulting midwife who never sees the client. This type of "hallway consultation" (Gottlieb, 2006) has limited application for clinical situations. The limitation of such consultation should be at the forefront of the midwife's mind. When tests are ordered, the results become an aspect of care that must be taken under consideration for further care. Implementing care without adequate understanding of lab results may waste valuable time and may even present unnecessary risk.

REFERENCES

Ament, L. A. (Ed.). (2007). *Professional issues in midwifery*. Sudbury, MA: Jones and Bartlett.

Ament, L. A., & Tillett, J. (2007). Quality management. In L. A. Ament (Ed.), *Professional issues in midwifery* (pp. 249–261). Sudbury, MA: Jones and Bartlett.

American College of Nurse-Midwives (ACNM). (1997). *Position statement: Certified nurse-midwives and certified midwives as primary care providers/case managers*. Retrieved January 26, 2009, from http://www.midwife.org/position.cfm

American College of Nurse-Midwives (ACNM). (2003). *Standards for the practice of midwifery*. Retrieved August 3, 2009, from http://www.midwife.org/siteFiles/descriptive/Standards_for_Practice _of_Midwifery_2003.pdf

American College of Nurse-Midwives (ACNM). (2005). *Position statement: quality management in midwifery care.* Retrieved from http://www.midwife.org/siteFiles/position/Quality _Management_05.pdf

American College of Nurse-Midwives (ACNM). (2007). *Core competencies for basic midwifery practice.* Retrieved August 3, 2009, from http://www.midwife.org/siteFiles/descriptive/Core _Competencies_6_07.pdf

American College of Nurse-Midwives (ACNM). (2008). *American College of Nurse-Midwives code of ethics with explanatory statements.* Silver Spring, MD: Author.

American Nurses Association (ANA). (2005). *Code of ethics for nurses.* Retrieved January 26, 2009, from http://nursingworld.org/ethics/code/protected_nwcoe813.htm

American Psychiatric Association (APA). (2000). *Diagnostic and statistical manual of mental disorders* (4th ed., text revision). Washington, DC: Author.

Beauchamp, T. L., & Childress, J. F. (2009). *Principles of biomedical ethics* (6th ed.). New York: Oxford University Press.

College of Midwives of British Columbia. (1996). *Code of ethics.* Retrieved January 26, 2009, from http://cmbc.bc.ca/MENU-Model-of-Care.shtml

Davis, E. (2004). *Heart and hands: A midwife's guide to pregnancy and birth.* Berkeley, CA: Celestial Arts.

Gottlieb, M. C. (2006). A template for peer ethics consultation. *Ethics & Behavior, 16*(2), 151–162.

International Confederation of Midwives (ICM). (2003). *ICM international code of ethics for midwives.* Retrieved January 30, 2009, from http://www.internationalmidwives.org/Documentation /Coredocuments/tabid/322/Default.aspx

Jacob, S., & Hartshorne, T. S. (2003). *Ethics and law for school psychologists.* Hoboken, NJ: Wiley.

McCool, W. F., & McCartney, M. (2007). Midwifery scope of practice. In L. A. Ament (Ed.), *Professional issues in midwifery* (pp. 175–190). Sudbury, MA: Jones and Bartlett.

Midwives Alliance of North America (MANA). (2005). *Standards and qualifications for the art and practice of midwifery.* Washington, DC: Author.

National Association of Certified Professional Midwives (NACPM). (2004). *Essential documents.* Retrieved August 1, 2009, from http://www.nacpm.org/Resources/nacpm-standards.pdf

North American Registry of Midwives (NARM). (2006). *NARM community peer review: Community peer review process.* Retrieved August 6, 2009, from http://www.narm.org/peerreview.htm

Nursing and Midwifery Council. (2002). Codes and declarations. *Nursing Ethics, 9*(6), 674–680.

Rooks, J. P. (2007). Relationships between CNMs and CMs and other midwives, nurses, and physicians. In L. A. Ament (Ed.), *Professional issues in midwifery* (pp. 1–40). Sudbury, MA: Jones and Bartlett.

Texas Midwifery Board. (2005). *Scope of practice.* Retrieved January 26, 2009, from http://www .dshs.state.tx.us/midwife/mw_scope.shtm

CHAPTER 8

Working with Other Professionals

Serving women and their families often requires consultation with other professionals. Whether the issue is related to mental health, a medical condition unrelated to pregnancy, or a cultural barrier, high-quality holistic care frequently involves collaboration or consultation with other midwives as well as professionals from other fields. The Midwives Model of Care (MMOC) (Rothman, 1979) supports midwives working within their scope of practice and developing relationships with other professionals while facilitating collaboration, consultation, and referral. In this respect, clinical and ethical standards converge.

> Community-based care requires that the clinician provide ongoing screening for problems or potential problems that may have an impact on perinatal outcome. When deviations from normal are identified, the clinician must determine whether clinical management can continue to be provided independently, whether consultation and/or collaboration is appropriate, or whether referral to an obstetric specialist is indicated. State regulations, professional organization policies and position statements, and the relationship between the midwife and other members of the prenatal health care team all must be considered when determining the appropriate level of management. Decisions regarding level of care must be made in collaboration with the woman and her family in a way that respects the cultural values and beliefs held in the family and community. (Walsh, 2001, p. 385)

Working within one's scope of practice and valuing the knowledge of other professionals are ethical components related to consultation and collaboration. When midwives operate within their scope of practice, they can provide high-quality care. However, midwives who stretch into areas beyond their knowledge and skill level can potentially do much harm. The best midwifery care involves a competent and skilled midwife who recognizes her limitations and defers to other knowledgeable professionals when appropriate (refer to Chapter 7 in this text for more information relating to scope of practice). Through the care of various professionals, women build trusting relationships with other healthcare providers who can continue providing care for them and their families beyond the childbearing years.

This chapter is different from other chapters in this book in that it does not focus on a particular ethical issue, such as informed consent. Rather, multiple ethical standards are related to the topic of working with other professionals. We begin by exploring relationships with other healthcare providers, including physicians, holistic practitioners, and other birth and lactation specialists. We consider how midwives relate to one another, including a section on bullying, which has been identified as commonplace among nurses and midwives (Hastie, 1996; Joint Commission, 2008; Stevens, 2002). Then we examine pertinent ethical issues in consultation, collaboration, referral, and transfer before providing case studies for consideration. For midwives to become central to maternity care in the United States, we must learn to work in relationship with other healthcare providers (Davis-Floyd & Johnson, 2006). Applied professional ethics can help us collaborate with these valuable human resources in our communities while maintaining the values related to the MMOC.

PHYSICIANS

Midwives, midwifery clients, and physicians all stand to benefit from collaborative work between midwives, physicians, and other medical professionals. Regrettably, many midwives are intimidated by physicians and avoid contact with them. It is likely that this attitude is related to the cultural marginalization of midwives in local healthcare systems and communities (see Chapter 1). Another divisive factor between midwives and doctors lies in their contrasting models of care, reliance on technology, and attitudes regarding birth. Despite these differences, midwives must take responsibility for bridging the gap in communication between themselves and physicians because it is essential for high-quality care. In so doing, a midwife must maintain her role in safeguarding her client from unethical practices.

Many midwives have daily contact and working relationships with doctors, whereas others rarely encounter physicians in their work with women. It stands to reason that if our clients can benefit from our own relationships with physicians, then it is our responsibility to attempt to build relationships with them. Physicians possess skills and expertise that can benefit women. Some specialists, such as obstetricians and perinatologists, have specialized knowledge related to maternity care. Although their expertise relates largely to pathology, their knowledge complements that of the midwife, an expert in healthy maternity care and normal birth. "Attention to the pathologic potential of pregnancy is vital because, although most pregnancies would proceed healthfully without any medical intervention, serious complications and diseases are not uncommon and can be deadly" (Rooks, 1999, p. 371). Midwifery care is largely complementary to medical care, with a significant degree of overlap between the two. High-quality maternity care in a community could not exist without the presence of both midwives and physicians.

Unfortunately, in many instances midwives and physicians lack good communication as a result of competitive, hierarchical, educational, and institutional barriers. This lack of communication is potentially detrimental both to midwives and physicians, as well as to the childbearing women whom they serve. Imagine a homebirth midwife who transports a client for a serious intrapartal complication, such as fetal distress. The quality of the client's care will largely relate to the smoothness in transition between midwifery and physician care. If the physician does not understand the midwife's role at the birth, dismisses her charting, or ignores her diagnosis, the client may be subjected to unnecessary risk or stressful procedures. The doctor may file a complaint against the midwife due to miscommunication even if she acted according to sound protocols. Conversely, the doctor may suffer a malpractice suit if he disregards vital information in the midwife's chart that could inform treatment. Communication gaps between midwives and physicians can be problematic for hospital and community practices.

In contrast, midwives who effectively collaborate with physicians build communication skills needed to achieve smooth transitions between care, and all parties stand to benefit. Clients benefit from professional standards of care. Their midwives may have privileges at hospitals or be welcome in hospital delivery rooms. Physicians are more likely to treat midwives with respect and seek their input when good communication is established. Further, physicians themselves benefit by building professional relationships with midwives who provide referral to their practices. "The physician/midwife relationship is mutually beneficial as the physician aligns him or herself with a source of referrals and the midwife develops a collegial relationship with a physician who is available for consultation and collaboration" (American College of Nurse-Midwives, 2005, p. 1).

Mary Barnett, CNM, who has considerable experience in both hospital and out-of-hospital midwifery practice, has concluded that it is essential for midwives to learn to communicate with physicians in medical language (personal communication, July 1, 2008). She advocates precise charting with language that matches that used by physicians. Whereas certified nurse–midwives (CNMs) are likely to attain mastery of medical terminology in nursing and nurse midwifery school, certified professional midwives (CPMs) must seek opportunities to expand their knowledge of medical language through study, conference seminars, or college classes if they did not obtain that knowledge during the midwifery educational process. Because midwives who seek physician collaboration or transfer are working on the physician's turf (i.e., the hospital or doctor's clinic), it behooves the midwife to take responsibility for bridging the gap of communication when referring clients to physicians. In the process she will diminish the Tower of Babel effect and promote understanding that will benefit her clients' care and her own relationships with other medical professionals.

Irrespective of the quality of the midwife-physician relationship, when midwives disagree with physicians' behaviors, it is imperative that they do not become complicit in unethical behavior. We are required by our professional values (and ethical codes) to uphold a woman's dignity, her right to informed choice, and her access to reproductive counseling and contraception. Further, we must uphold principles of nonmaleficence and beneficence and, in so doing, assist women in avoiding potentially dangerous or unnecessary interventions (Thompson & Thompson, 1997). Chapter 11 discusses ways to address ethical conflicts, including disagreements concerning the behaviors of others. Effective communication with physicians is of paramount importance for midwives to provide optimal care to clients. The same holds true with other health professionals.

COMPLEMENTARY AND ALTERNATIVE MEDICINE PROFESSIONALS

Even midwives who do not identify with complementary and alternative medicine (CAM) encounter women who seek naturopathic remedies or some other nonallopathic healthcare modality with which the midwife has little expertise. "Enabling women to use complementary and alternative therapies empowers them in the childbearing process and provides them with additional resources, which are not only therapeutically effective but also often relaxing and calming" (Tiran, 2004, p. 338). Professional acupuncturists, herbalists, massage therapists, and naturopaths are among the many types of alternative healthcare practitioners sought by women during the childbirth year.

Many midwives incorporate the use of herbal, homeopathic, and other alternative or traditional medicines in their practices. As with allopathic (conventional) medicine, training and knowledge in these modalities, informed choice, and attention to evidence-based practice are required for responsible ethical care. Yet, there are many appropriate times for referral to a professional alternative healthcare practitioner. Most of these modalities are discrete fields requiring advanced degrees to practice, and working without adequate training in these areas may result in harm to clients (Tiran, 2004). "The majority of decision-making in CAM is based on experience, observation and traditional healing manuscripts" (Mills, Hollyer, Saranchuk, & Wilson, 2002, p. 1). Hence, it may be difficult for midwives to achieve the required knowledge and skills in CAM. Midwives who wish to work in depth in one of these areas should seek additional education and training as required to provide competent care (see Chapter 7). Indeed, some midwives obtain licensure or certification as acupuncturists, massage therapists, or yoga instructors.

Some clients have personal knowledge and experience with home remedies. With the proliferation and increased accessibility of information concerning holistic healthcare practices, women are increasingly gaining knowledge of these practices and are incorporating them into their personal and family health care. For the midwife, keeping up with these trends presents challenges. One may not have experience with the home remedies clients are using. This situation requires, at the least, time to adequately research remedies and, ideally, access to herbalists, as well as naturopathic and homeopathic doctors, for consultation, referral, and collaboration. Developing relationships in one's community with these providers will enhance your practice and assist you in building professional networks.

As part of the ethical principle of nonmaleficence, a midwife should not recommend alternative therapies that are potentially harmful. It follows that she should not recommend therapies of which she has little or no knowledge, that are not evidence based, or that are experimental. Likewise, she should avoid recommendation to a care provider for whom she feels little confidence or trust. When a midwife works with other professionals in the holistic healthcare movement, she is entrusting her clients to the knowledge and practice of those clinicians. Her clients trust her judgment and will often follow the advice of those whom she recommends. Building relationships with alternative healthcare providers in her area will help ensure that her clients receive the best care. For additional information on this subject, see the discussion of collaborative care later in this chapter.

In summary, when a client can benefit from consultation, collaboration, or referral to an alternative healthcare specialist, the midwife serves an important role in facilitating these relationships. Before making a referral, the midwife must determine that the provider is competent and appropriate for her client. Midwives can learn how to serve their clients better by developing good working relationships with CAM providers.

OTHER BIRTH AND BREASTFEEDING PROFESSIONALS

Midwifery care is enhanced by working with other birth and breastfeeding specialists. Frequently, a midwife consults or collaborates with other midwives to improve the care that she delivers. Clients are likely to have better outcomes when another professional is brought in for appropriate supplemental care, whether it be by their request or the midwife's referral.

Perhaps the most common form of consultation in midwifery practice is between a midwife and her peers. Whether working alone in private practice or in a group setting, midwives often consult with one another about their clients. When doing so, it is imperative that midwives maintain confidentiality (see Chapter 3). Through consultation with other midwives, a midwife often gains insight into her cases. Numerous contextual factors lead to the midwife seeking a consultation. New midwives may encounter situations that other midwives have experienced. One way to improve one's care is to seek expert consultation from a seasoned midwife when these situations arise. Sometimes midwives consult one another to see different perspectives on a situation, to seek validation for a decision, or to share the joys and disappointments of clinical experiences. Midwives also collaborate with and refer to one another in providing care to women. Midwives are a valuable source of social and professional support for one another. For this reason, it is imperative that midwives work to sustain healthy communication and professional behavior among themselves.

Midwives provide comprehensive care, and although most midwifery clients do not need the assistance of another birth or breastfeeding professional, some situations require additional services. When women lack social resources, other professionals provide much-needed social support during critical periods. Consider the service of doulas. The presence of a birth doula can make a big difference in the outcome of a long birth, and the presence of a postpartum doula is frequently required for the care of newborn twins. Doulas provide social support for women in the childbearing year that goes beyond that typically provided by a midwife. Usually, the doula's skills are greater than those of an untrained family member because the doula is an authoritative source of information on birth, lactation, and newborn care. Some clients request the presence of a doula at their births or in the postpartum period. There are other types of birth and lactation professionals that a midwife may need to access for her practice. Perhaps a midwife encounters a breastfeeding challenge with which she has little expertise, and the help of a lactation consultant is required. Additionally, a midwife may refer her clients to a childbirth educator for birthing classes.

When we find ourselves working with other maternity and lactation specialists, ethical considerations arise. One ethical issue that we have already related to this chapter is scope of practice. When the midwife has exhausted her knowledge in a given area, such as breastfeeding, and the client's problem persists, it is time to consult, collaborate, or refer to a specialist. Similarly, when a midwife does not provide a service, such as childbirth classes, and the client either requests or can benefit from such a service, it is time to refer. Midwives should share information with other birth professionals on a need-to-know basis and maintain confidentiality. Finally, midwives must extend respect to other professionals.

RELATIONSHIPS AMONG MIDWIVES

In considering relationships among midwives, it is necessary to reflect on the history between direct-entry midwives (DEMs) and nurse–midwives in the United States. Specifically, we focus on the relationship between the Midwives Alliance of North America (MANA) and the American College of Nurse-Midwives (ACNM), the two most prominent organizations representing midwives in the United States. There is a long history of successful collaboration between ACNM and MANA, as well as areas of significant conflict (Davis-Floyd & Johnson, 2006; Geradine Simkins, personal communication, July 14, 2009).

The primary source of division between the two organizations lies in their differing opinions on midwifery training and education. At one time, ACNM viewed nursing to be the only route to becoming a qualified midwife. Now, ACNM has its own direct-entry certification, the CM, which was developed at the same time that MANA was introducing its DEM certification, the CPM. At the date of this writing, there are approximately 65 CMs and over 1,500 CPMs (Geradine Simkins, personal communication, July 14, 2009).

ACNM holds the position that graduation from a formal education program, typically a college or university-based midwifery course of study, is the only bona fide educational route to becoming a DEM. MANA, on the other hand, supports multiple routes of entry into the profession of midwifery, including competency-based training and education through enrollment at a midwifery school or a college-based educational program (Geradine Simkins, personal communication, July 14, 2009). Both the CPM and the CM are nationally accredited midwifery credentials.

Rather than focusing on differences, midwives can better serve their profession and childbearing women through unified efforts to integrate midwifery into mainstream maternity care (Davis-Floyd & Johnson, 2006). MANA's Bridge Club and Sister Angela Murdaugh's efforts are among those that have brought CPMs and CNMs together collegially. Conversely, when midwives quarrel among themselves, it reflects poorly on the profession.

In an effort to promote harmony and respect among diverse midwives, The Bridge Club was formed in the 1990s (MANA, 2009). Open to students and midwives with a wide range of credentials, The Bridge Club has grown to over 200 members. Meetings are held annually at the MANA and ACNM conferences, and an Internet discussion group has formed to encourage dialogue. The group's energy is directed toward building connections between midwives and promoting unity and understanding.

Sister Angela Murdaugh, ACNM President (1981–1982), organized The Gathering of Texas Midwives in 1997, a conscious effort to bring midwives together for "a fun weekend and CEUs" (continuing education credits). Held annually, The

Gathering of Texas Midwives hosts CPMs and CNMs to learn together, celebrate midwifery, and honor one another. One of the highlights of the weekend is Sister Angela's blessing of the hands. "People are people," says Sister Angela, "when you get to know them. We can agree to disagree, but try to understand everyone's point of view and find common ground, making a human connection." The Gathering of Midwives is an opportunity to renew spirit in multiple ways. Sister Angela views diversity in midwifery as an asset to the public and individuals who have different needs. "We don't have to be united, but we have to be respectful" (personal communication, October 15, 2009).

Bullying

The midwifery community should be a haven of sisterhood and support for its practitioners. After all, we are a minority group working within a hierarchically structured healthcare industry where physicians and hospital administrators hold the majority of the power at the top. Many of us are disenfranchised from our local healthcare communities. We are typically women serving women in a woman-centered manner, working exhausting hours, often at the expense of our own families. More than a few of us identify with feminism. Ironically, midwives do not always treat one another with dignity and respect. Midwives are becoming increasingly aware of the extent to which bullying has become a professional concern (Farrell, 2006, 2007; Gillen, Sinclair, & Kernohan, 2004; Hadikin, 2001). The bulk of the scholarly articles and books on the topic originate from New Zealand and the United Kingdom. Even so, U.S. midwives have also reported bullying, and some believe that it is a systemic problem in our field (Farrell, 2006).

People who bully often feel threatened and are resistant to change (Farrell, 2007). Overt monitoring, humiliating, persistently criticizing, spreading malicious rumors, and excluding or ignoring are common bullying behaviors (Hadikin, 2001). In addition to individuals' behaviors, hierarchical structures may support bullying, much to the detriment of the quality of midwifery care (Hollins Martin & Bull, 2006). Hastie (1996) argues that horizontal violence (i.e., when midwives bully one another) is a contextual phenomenon that originates from the dominant hegemony, the oppression of women. Theoretically, members of disenfranchised groups attempt to establish hierarchical structures to protect themselves through aggressive behavior.

Bullying can have devastating effects on victims, inducing stress-related disorders and interference with job performance (Hadikin, 2001). "Intimidating and disruptive behaviors can foster medical errors, contribute to poor patient satisfaction and to preventable adverse outcomes, increase the cost of care, and cause qualified clinicians, administrators and managers to seek new positions in more professional environments" (Joint Commission, 2008, n.p.).

The ethical principles of beneficence, nonmaleficence, autonomy, and justice do not apply exclusively to the midwife-client relationship; midwives must apply these same principles when working with other professionals, including midwifery colleagues. It is a great travesty to the profession when new, educated, inspired midwives are discredited and undermined by those who are threatened by shifting ways and ideas.

To overcome these dynamics, midwifery organizations must take a stand on professional behavior among midwives. Midwifery organizations can explore the concept of the integrity of the healthcare professional and create codes of conduct that set parameters on the behavior of midwives regarding their relationships with others (Aiken, 2009). Midwives must not tolerate bullying in their labor and delivery units or their community. To stop bullying behavior, an individual or group must confront the perpetrator or perpetrators, explain the effects of their behavior, and ask them to stop (Hadikin, 2001). Bullying is damaging to the bully, the victim, the community, and the profession. Greater awareness of bullying and codes of professional conduct that focus on professional relationships are needed.

THE CODES

The existing ethical codes have some general guidelines regarding collaboration, referral, and transfer of care. Some emphasize ethics in relationships with other professionals. We here consider the International Code of Ethics for Midwives written by the International Confederation of Midwives (ICM, 2003), the Code of Ethics of ACNM (2008), the Statement of Values and Ethics of MANA (1997), and the Essential Documents of the National Association of Certified Professional Midwives (NACPM, 2004). We also examine the Codes and Declarations of the Nursing and Midwifery Council (NMC, 2002). Each of these documents can be found in the appendices. Finally, we look at the Code of Ethics for Nurses with Interpretive Statements of the American Nurses Association (ANA, 2001).

Among the midwifery codes, ICM's International Code of Ethics for Midwives (2003; see Appendix D) contains the most developed guidelines relating to working with other professionals. Prominently, the first section of the code is entitled "Midwifery Relationships" and includes the following statement: "Midwives support and sustain each other in their professional roles, and actively nurture their own and others' sense of self-worth" (p. 1). This statement clearly addresses professional relationships among midwives. It is a declaration that midwives must work to support and validate one another.

A related statement provides further instruction: "Midwives recognise the human interdependence within their field of practice and actively seek to solve inherent conflicts" (ICM, 2003, p. 1). ICM further elaborates on this statement in the section "Glossary of Terms Used in the ICM International Code of Ethics for Midwives." For the term *human interdependence*, ICM writes:

> Since midwives work in relationship with women and others and may not always agree about what is right or should be done in a given situation, it is important that midwives seek to understand the reasons for the disagreements with clients or colleagues. Midwives do not stop with understanding or respect, however. They also work to resolve those conflicts that need to be resolved in order for ethical care to continue. (p. 3)

The attention devoted to the concept of human interdependence in the glossary underlines the emphasis ICM places on relationships. Specifically, we are instructed by this definition to go beyond quelling disagreements and to actively seek resolution of conflict and disagreements with clients or colleagues.

In relation to consultation and referral, ICM states, "Midwives work with other health professionals, consulting and referring as necessary when the woman's need for care exceeds the competencies of the midwife" (ICM, 2003, p. 1). This is a general statement summarizing the midwife's ethical responsibility to seek expert consultation or to refer a client when "necessary." The vagueness of the term *necessary* may be purposeful, so as not to limit or define the scope of practice of international midwives, whose local jurisdictions may have more to say about the areas of competency in midwifery. However, the vague nature of the statement does not weaken its message that midwives consult and refer when appropriate, keeping within their areas of competency.

The final statement in ICM's code related to working with others involves privacy: "Midwives hold in confidence client information in order to protect the right to privacy, and use judgment in sharing this information" (ICM, 2003, p. 2). When working with other professionals, midwives exercise judgment in sharing a client's information with other care providers.

Now we turn to ACNM's input regarding work with other professionals. ACNM (2008) offers guidance regarding relationships in terms of autonomy and dignity in its Code of Ethics with Explanatory Statements (see Appendix C). Strong language is utilized throughout:

> [Respecting human dignity] requires midwives to listen to, recognize and reflect on different points of view to understand any impact these differences may have on

the professional relationship and the choices and outcomes of care . . . This moral obligation applies to all persons with whom midwives have professional relationships, including those who receive midwifery care, members of the health-care team, administrators, policy makers and students. Trust, integrity, truth-telling, compassion, caring, and respect form the foundation for positive professional relationships. (pp. 3–4)

Further guidance to protect against harmful practices relates to the ethical principles of nonmaleficence and beneficence. ACNM requires its members to prevent harmful practices and intervene when they occur.

In contrast, the Essential Documents of NACPM (2004; see Appendix E) does not address collegial relationships specifically. Attention to collaboration and referral is presented in the context of safety for women and newborns. The NACPM member makes appropriate referrals when the client's needs are out of his or her scope of practice, collaborates with other providers, and maintains support for women when transfer of care is required.

Like ICM's code, MANA's (1997) Statement of Values and Ethics (Appendix A) includes a section on relationships. The wording reflects values and does not describe behavior. Far from ACNM's (2008) position, there are no ethical requirements in relationships with others. The values in relationships include honesty, mutual trust, and respect. More specifically for midwives, MANA states that "we value the midwifery community as a support system and an essential place for learning and sisterhood" (1997, p. 4).

Other codes that may not apply specifically to U.S. midwives provide valuable insight and guidance with respect to relationships with other professionals. For example, the Codes and Declarations of the Nursing and Midwifery Council of the United Kingdom (2002; see Appendix F) contains a more descriptive code of professional conduct. This is similar to other applied fields in the United States (e.g., the American Psychological Association, 2003). Likewise, the American Nurses Association's Code of Ethics for Nurses with Interpretive Statements (2001) includes a significant section devoted to the topic of professional relationships with colleagues and contains specified behavioral components:

The principle of respect for persons extends to all individuals with whom the nurse interacts. The nurse maintains compassionate and caring relationships with colleagues and others with a commitment to the fair treatment of individuals, to integrity-preserving compromise, and to resolving conflict . . . the nurse treats colleagues, employees, assistants, and students with respect and compassion. This standard of conduct precludes all prejudicial actions, any form of harassment or threatening behavior, or disregard for the effect of one's actions on others. The nurse values the distinctive contribution of individuals or groups, and collaborates to meet the shared goal of providing quality health services. (ANA, 2001, n.p.)

COLLABORATIVE CARE

Many women who employ midwives also seek the services of other professionals. Chiropractors, medical doctors, naturopaths, and other professionals often serve women who are under the care of midwives simultaneously. Although there is nothing inherently unethical about such arrangements, the potential for ethical concerns exists, and midwives are advised to be aware of possible risks so that efforts can be made to minimize harm.

One area of concern that can emerge is conflicting recommendations, which can result in client confusion and perhaps stress. Additionally, the client who decides to follow the recommendations of both the midwife and the other practitioner could put herself at greater risk for health problems. For example, an expectant mother is seeing a massage therapist who recommends exercises to relieve low-back pain. Yet, the exercises are inappropriate for pregnancy and can exacerbate lordosis. The midwife has an ethical obligation of beneficence; therefore, the midwife must intervene if she learns of bad advice that is placing her client at risk. Her obligation is to address the issue directly with the client, instructing her to avoid inappropriate movements in pregnancy, and offering safe alternatives when possible. The midwife has no ethical obligation to the massage therapist, but offering her instructive feedback may be appropriate if a professional relationship exists between the two care providers.

When a client shares with her midwife that she receives services from other professionals, the midwife should inform the client of the benefits and risks of coordinated care and recommend that the client consent to a release of information between the two (or more) providers (see Chapter 4). When a client gives a midwife and other providers consent to communicate with one another about the client's care, each professional can work in concert with the other providers to avoid duplication of services or contradictory practices. Furthermore, the specialist's care may be highly informed by the midwife's perspective on the client's pregnancy. This is common when women are referred to physicians, acupuncturists, massage therapists, and chiropractors. Midwives can include information in their privacy statements that explains how client records are shared with other healthcare professionals in instances of collaborative care. Midwives cannot assume that clients will read privacy statements closely, so a verbal explanation is often necessary to ensure comprehension of privacy policies.

TRANSFER OF CARE

Transfer of care to another midwife or a physician may be indicated in a variety of situations. Six months into her pregnancy a client may develop a complication, such as preeclampsia, that requires a physician's care. Alternatively, a midwife may become ill and unable to practice, thereby needing to facilitate a transfer of care for her clients to another care provider. When such transfers occur, they should be done responsibly and in accordance with ethical and legal standards. ACNM's Code of Ethics with Explanatory Statements (2008) notes that midwives unable to continue care attempt to provide "seamless transfer of care" for those they serve.

Midwives should make every effort to facilitate transfer of care with the client's needs in mind. Optimally, transitioning from one provider to another should be seamless and not leave a gap in the client's care. For example, a midwife's client is found to be carrying twins at 20 weeks. The midwife does not feel that twins are within her scope of practice. She is aware of other midwives who provide care for twins, and many doctors in town will willingly accept her client at 20 weeks. Optimally, the midwife can act as a guide and provide the client with opportunities to meet other providers so as to avoid any form of abandonment, as well as to help smooth the transition for all involved parties.

REFERRAL AND CONSULTATION

A midwife should refer a client to another care provider when the client has a problem that is beyond the midwife's competency, when a client can benefit from referral, or at the client's request. "Consultation refers to the situation where a midwife recommends the woman consult a medical practitioner, or when a woman requests another opinion of a medical practitioner" (Tracy & Miller, 2006, pp. 275–276). Midwives seek consultation when a complication arises in the course of a woman's care, unless transfer is required. Consultation may be with a midwife or physician, but CAM providers may also be consultants to midwives and their clients. At the outset, the client should be notified that consultation is warranted. The midwife has the responsibility to initiate the consultation, but the client and the consultant are included in decisions made regarding clinical roles and responsibilities, collaborative care, or a transfer of care (Tracy & Miller, 2006). In some situations, a client may refuse consultation, which can open up other ethical considerations (see Chapter 9 for information about client noncompliance).

In addition to client consultation, midwives often seek professional consultation with one another or other healthcare providers for professional advice. This type of communication, sometimes called peer-to-peer consultation, occurs when a midwife calls a colleague about a client for advice regarding interpretation of labs and clinical finding as well as the development of a plan of care. In these cases, the midwife must exercise caution in implementing advice from another healthcare professional who has not personally evaluated the client. Further vigilance is advised in sharing privacy information with anyone who is not directly involved in the client's care.

Referring a client for a service may be difficult when a midwife fears that she may appear incompetent or lose the client. This has been discussed in the field of dentistry, but the concept can be applied to other professions (Steier & Steier, 2008). In midwifery, some expertise among providers is apparent in clinical skill, experience, and scope of practice. A midwife who has never assisted a breech delivery, for example, is not able to serve such a client as well as one who has vast experience with this fetal position in labor and birth. The primary midwife may feel uncertain as to whether her client will identify more with the more experienced colleague, but the clinician's fears must not bear on the decision to refer, consult, or collaborate in care.

Referral must be free of remuneration as a result of referral to another care provider. Remuneration (informally known as "kickbacks") creates a conflict of interest and impairs the clinician's ability to best serve the client's needs. Beckwith (1996) addresses this issue in the context of health maintenance organization (HMO) practices in which the primary care physician receives kickbacks by not making referrals. Rowdin (as cited in Beckwith, 1996) argues that "incentives also undermine other practices, such as informed consent" (p. 153). The American College of Physicians (1998) has addressed this issue in detail, restricting physicians from fee-splitting that results from referral to another physician, as well as any form of commission or kickback. When midwives refer to other healthcare providers, they must be aware of conflicting interests and put the client's needs above all others.

Ethical practice with other professionals requires knowledge, honesty, diplomacy, and respect. One may not begin her practice with all of these skills intact, and most will falter on occasion. Studying ethics is a first step in successful ethical practice. Being mindful of one's own motives and limitations can assist the development of ethical behavior towards colleagues. Maintaining healthy relationships with other providers is essential to uphold the integrity of the profession of midwifery.

CASE EXAMPLES

CASE 1

Emily is a new midwife at a small community birth center. She is a recent graduate and is very enthusiastic about woman-centered midwifery care. She eagerly participates in all levels of involvement at the birth center, and frequently offers her input and ideas to the group of midwives with whom she works.

Some of the midwives who have been working at the birth center for a while find Emily's enthusiasm to be amusing and even inspiring at times. They often listen to Emily's ideas and offer genuine feedback and support. However, Felicia and Joan find Emily's exuberance annoying and naive. Together, they attempt to discredit Emily, often being overly critical of her work, discrediting her credentials, and excluding her whenever possible.

Emily reacts by trying harder to gain approval: putting in longer hours and taking on challenging projects. She even offers to take call for other midwives when they need assistance or time off. Joan and Felicia see her deepening level of dedication as threatening to their jobs and the status quo. They do not wish to work longer hours to keep pace with the new midwife. They begin gossiping about her to other midwives at the center.

Questions

1. Which ethical principles and codes are relevant to this case?
2. How are the dynamics of the case relevant to bullying?
3. How should the other midwives at the birth center react to the conflict?

Analysis

The case of Emily, Felicia, and Joan illustrates a typical bullying situation in nursing and midwifery. A new, creative, and inspired midwife meets resistance from peers and superiors and eventually becomes the target of bullying. Her perpetrators use bullying strategies to disempower and discredit her in order to maintain power structures and the status quo. If this pattern continues, Emily's health and job performance may suffer. She may leave the profession out of frustration and fear. Her community and the profession of midwifery stand to suffer should the bullying continue.

Respect for the dignity of others is perhaps the most salient ethical issue in this case. All human beings are deserving of dignity, and to treat someone with utter contempt and attempt to harm that person, either personally or professionally, is a threat to his or her dignity. Midwives should respect dignity and avoid bullying.

The ethical principle of nonmaleficence prohibits a midwife from bullying because bullying poses harm to another person. It is not acceptable to harm a colleague. The ethical codes that specifically address this issue include ANA's Code of Ethics for Nurses (2001), ICM's International Code of Ethics for Midwives (2003), and, to a lesser degree, ACNM's Code of Ethics (2008). Felicia and Joan's behavior requires intervention from another midwife to stop the bullying. The ethical principle of beneficence requires midwives to protect others from harm. The midwives at the birth center who witness the bullying are thus ethically responsible to intervene.

A hierarchical structure may be the root cause of the bullying problem. As midwives compete for powerful positions, those at the top may become abusive as a means to maintain their power, whereas those with the least amount of power are vulnerable to bullying tactics. This social psychological phenomenon was best illustrated by the Stanford prison experiment (Zimbardo, 1971), an infamous study entrenched in debate over the ethical treatment of human subjects. Zimbardo's study illustrates the disturbing effects that roles play in shaping human behavior. Studies conducted in the United Kingdom demonstrate that situational factors, including fear of conflict, intimidation, litigation, and consequences from challenging senior staff, as well as an obligation to follow hospital policies, affected obedient behavior among midwives, who abandoned woman-centered care in order to avoid punishment (Hollins Martin & Bull, 2006). Therefore, it is essential that the workplace be free of intimidation so that midwives can do the work they were trained to do: provide woman-centered care. The administrators at the birth center may need to examine their organizational structure to ascertain the need to reorganize or adopt a cooperative model or policies that prohibit bullying.

Case 2

Helen is a midwife in an urban private practice adjacent to a hospital with a busy labor and delivery floor where she comes into contact with numerous doctors and nurses. Her practice is one of only two midwifery practices with privileges at the facility. She values woman-centered maternity care, but often feels pressured by the hospital nurses to toe the line and abide by standard practices and hospital policies regarding procedures such as external fetal monitoring (EFM), amniotomy, and nutritional restrictions.

One of Helen's clients arrived at the hospital in early labor with a breech presentation, and an obstetrician was called in to collaborate care. Dr. Wang and Helen had worked together in the past when complications arose during antenatal care, but this was the first labor complication that she'd experienced on his call. Helen was aware that most doctors in her community did not deliver breeches vaginally, although many out-of-hospital midwives did. Helen had assisted with a few breeches in her training and practice prior to moving to her current location. She felt that her client was a good candidate for breech vaginal delivery. She discussed her perspective with Dr. Wang.

Dr. Wang did not attend breech vaginal births, and was unwilling to begin doing so with a midwife's client. He expressed his professional opinion that cesarean section was safest. Helen acquiesced without pushing further, and told her client that surgical delivery was her only option. The client became emotional and began to protest, and Dr. Wang came in to explain the risks of vaginal delivery of a breech. He did not mention the risks of the surgery or other alternatives. Although Helen disagreed with Dr. Wang's approach to patient counseling, she did not interrupt or challenge him. Instead, she focused on comforting her client and preparing her for the surgery.

Questions

1. How effective was the collaboration between Dr. Wang and Helen?
2. How well did the care providers meet the client's needs?
3. Did Helen have other options?

Analysis

Helen and Dr. Wang were able to discuss their different perspectives on the case. Dr. Wang maintained firm boundaries regarding his protocol of surgical delivery for all breeches. Because he was the specialist who was called in, he had more power in the decision-making process than did Helen. Helen supported Dr. Wang's decision without challenge, and did not attempt to offer further counseling than Dr. Wang offered to the client. In this way, the collaboration went smoothly, but there was a hidden cost.

Another physician might have been willing to supervise a breech delivery with Helen maintaining primary care of the client. Had Helen tried to call in someone else, she might have threatened the relationship between Dr. Wang and herself. However, her ethical responsibility to her client remains her main concern. In her discussion with Dr. Wang, Helen could have asked if another doctor were available who assisted vaginal breech births. She might have expressed to him her own experience with breech delivery.

Clearly, the client was displeased with her lack of choices. She might have felt more empowered had she been given informed choice. Was the doctor's concern about safety and protocols more important than the client's right to make informed choices? Obstetrical decisions are often made by physicians in an effort to protect themselves from malpractice suits (defensive medicine). Midwives have to balance the policies and needs of the various professionals with the needs of clients, while prioritizing those of the client. Helen decided to focus on meeting her client's adjustment needs, rather than make waves to attempt to give her a vaginal birth. This may have been the best choice she felt she could make at the time, but compromising a client's care for the sake of policy must not go unexamined. A local peer review would be an appropriate means to evaluate her actions.

CASE 3

Jill is a Floridian midwife with a diverse clinical population. On her initial visit, her new client reports a history of childhood sexual abuse. Maria is a primigravida client of Cuban descent. She has some physical and emotional manifestations of post-traumatic stress disorder (PTSD), including insomnia and anxiety. She is not currently under medical treatment, and she has never had therapy for the abuse she experienced as a young child, although she did seek spiritual guidance through her priest.

Jill is familiar with the research on the effects of sexual abuse on the childbearing year, and suggests that Maria seek therapy to assist her in her adjustment to pregnancy as well as her preparation for birth and parenthood. Maria resists seeing a therapist because "the abuse happened a long time ago and is no longer a problem." Jill charts Maria's refusal to get counseling, and commences routine prenatal care.

On the next prenatal visit, Maria shares her fears with Jill. She reports feeling fearful for her baby. She worries that her partner might try to molest the baby, although he is not a sexual perpetrator. Jill attempts to reassure Maria that her baby is safe, but feels at a loss about what else she can do for her client. She queries Maria about her openness to counseling, and suggests that the fears, insomnia, and anxiety may be linked to her earlier abuse.

Jill asks Maria directly about her resistance to therapy, and learns a great deal. Maria wants to protect her family. She is worried about revealing too much about the abuse and getting the perpetrator in trouble. Her parents are immigrants, and the extended family is a very tight-knit unit and protective of family secrets. Jill suggests that a Cuban therapist would understand her family needs. When Maria agrees to give therapy a try, Jill finds a therapist with expertise in healing sexual abuse.

The therapist, Juanita, begins meeting with Maria for weekly appointments in midpregnancy. She works with the midwife and Maria to develop coping strategies and communication cues for the birth. Jill provides relevant information about pregnancy, labor, and the postpartum period to Juanita to help her understand Maria's needs during each stage of the childbearing year. They continue to collaborate until after the birth, although Maria continues to see Juanita to begin to heal her emotional wounds.

Questions

1. What appropriate actions did the midwife take in referring this client?
2. What precautions are required when sharing privacy information with another professional when collaborating care?
3. How was Maria's care enhanced by the collaboration of her midwife and therapist?

Analysis

The midwife in this case determined early in care that a referral was appropriate to the situation. Although Maria had gone to her priest at some point to heal from her sexual abuse, she had not undergone therapy. The midwife was aware that unresolved issues surrounding sexual abuse could resurface during the childbearing year (Simkin & Klaus, 2004). When the client did not act on the first referral, Jill charted the refusal appropriately. As her client began displaying signs of PTSD, Jill persisted in exploring the client's resistance to therapy and was able to help Maria seek therapy. Sensitive to Maria's need to relate to a therapist who could understand her culture, Jill found an appropriate provider with competency in sexual abuse trauma. The midwife handled the referral both sensitively and professionally.

Over the course of Maria's care, the midwife and therapist communicated effectively regarding Maria's needs and coping strategies. This collaborative effort assisted Maria's adjustment to pregnancy and preparation for labor. Information about the therapeutic relationship was helpful for the midwife in supporting her client. In turn, the therapeutic relationship between Juanita and Maria was informed by the midwife's knowledge of women's needs in pregnancy and labor.

When the midwife has obtained the client's permission to share private information with other healthcare providers involved in her care, she is able to work with others in this collaborative manner, sharing information on a need-to-know basis. It is important to obtain written consent in the form of a HIPAA acknowledgement or other such form prior to sharing private information with another provider. This protects clients' confidentiality and respect for their autonomy in deciding with whom their records should be shared.

REFERENCES

Aiken, T. D. (2009). *Legal and ethical issues in health occupations* (2nd ed.). New Orleans, LA: Elsevier.

American College of Nurse-Midwives (ACNM). (2005). *Principles for equitable compensation agreements between midwives and physicians.* Retrieved July 7, 2009, from http://www.midwife.org /siteFiles/position/Principles_for_Equitable_Compensation_Agreements_05.pdf

American College of Nurse-Midwives (ACNM). (2008). *American College of Nurse-Midwives code of ethics with explanatory statements.* Silver Spring, MD: ACNM Ethics Committee.

American College of Physicians. (1998). Ethics manual: Fourth edition. *Annals of Internal Medicine, 128*(7), 576–594. Retrieved July 7, 2009, from http://www.annals.org/cgi/content/full/128/7/576

American Nurses Association (ANA). (2001). *Code of ethics for nurses with interpretive statements.* Retrieved July 7, 2009, from http://nursingworld.org/MainMenuCategories/Ethics Standards/CodeofEthics.aspx

American Psychological Association (APA). (2003). *Ethical principles of psychologists and code of conduct.* Retrieved July 7, 2009, from http://www.apa.org/ethics/code2002.html#intro

Beckwith, F. J. (1996). The ethics of referral kickbacks and self-referral and the HMO physician as gatekeeper: An ethical analysis. *Journal of Social Psychology, 27*(3), 41–48.

Davis-Floyd, R. E., & Johnson, C. B. (2006). *Mainstreaming midwives: The politics of change.* New York: Routledge.

Farrell, M. V. (2006). Bullying. *Midwifery Today, 80.* Retrieved October 29, 2009, from http://www.midwiferytoday.com/articles/bullying_1.asp

Farrell, M. V. (2007). Who is the bully? *Midwifery Today, 81.* Retrieved October 29, 2009, from http://www.midwiferytoday.com/articles/bullying_2.asp

Gillen, P., Sinclair, M., & Kernohan, G. (2004). A concept analysis of bullying in midwifery. *Evidence Based Midwifery, 2*(2), 46–51.

Hadikin, R. (2001). Workplace bullying in midwifery. *Midwives Information and Resource Service (MIDIRS), 11*(3). Retrieved July 7, 2009, from http://www.dreamcoach.co.uk/MIDIRS.htm

Hastie, C. (1996). Dying for the cause. *Australian College of Midwives Incorporated Journal, 9*(1), 28–30.

Hollins Martin, C. J., & Bull, P. (2006). What features of the maternity unit promote obedient behaviour from midwives? *Clinical Effectiveness in Nursing, 9*(2), 221–231.

International Confederation of Midwives (ICM). (2003). *ICM international code of ethics for midwives.* Retrieved January 30, 2009, from http://www.internationalmidwives.org/Documentation /Coredocuments/tabid/322/Default.aspx

The Joint Commission. (2008). Behaviors that undermine a culture of safety. *Sentinel Event, 40.* Retrieved October 19, 2009, from http://www.jointcommission.org/SentinelEvents/SentinelEvent Alert/sea_40.htm

Midwives Alliance of North America (MANA). (1997). *Statement of values and ethics.* Washington, DC: Author.

Midwives Alliance of North America (MANA). (2009). *MANA-ACNM Bridge Club.* Retrieved October 15, 2009, from http://mana.org/bridgeclub.html

Mills, E., Hollyer, T., Saranchuk, R., & Wilson, K. (2002). Teaching evidence-based complementary and alternative medicine (EBCAM); changing behaviours in the face of reticence: A cross-over trial. *BMC Medical Education, 2*, 1–6. Retrieved from http://www.biomedcentral.com/1472-6920/2/2

National Association of Certified Professional Midwives (NACPM). (2004). *Essential documents of the National Association of Certified Professional Midwives.* Retrieved July 7, 2009, from http://www.nacpm.org/Resources/nacpm-standards.pdf

Nursing and Midwifery Council. (2002). *Codes and declarations.* Retrieved July 7, 2009, from http://nej.sagepub.com/cgi/pdf_extract/9/6/674

Rooks, J. P. (1999). The midwifery model of care. *Journal of Nurse-Midwifery, 44*(4), 370–374.

Rothman, B. K. (1979). *Two models in maternity care: Defining and negotiating reality.* New York: New York University Press.

Simkin, P., & Klaus, P. (2004). *When survivors give birth: Understanding and healing the effects of early sexual abuse on childbearing women.* Seattle, WA: Woman Classic Day Publishing.

Steier, L., & Steier, G. (2008). The ethics of referral. *Private Dentistry,* 86–88.

Stevens, S. (2002). Nursing workforce retention: Challenging a bullying culture. *Health Affairs, 21*(5), 189–193.

Thompson, J. E., & Thompson, H. O. (1997). Ethics and midwifery practice. *World Health, 50*(2), 14–15.

Tiran, D. (2004). Complementary therapies in childbearing. In C. Henderson & S. MacDonald (Eds.), *Mayes midwifery.* Edinburgh, Scotland: Bailliere.

Tracy, S. K., & Miller, S. (2006). Working in collaboration. In S. Pairman, J. Pincombe, C. Thorogood, & S. K. Tracy (Eds.), *Midwifery: Preparation for practice.* Edinburgh, Scotland: Churchill Livingstone.

Walsh, L. V. (2001). *Midwifery: Community based care during the childbearing year.* Philadelphia: W. B. Saunders.

Zimbardo, P. G. (1971). The power and pathology of imprisonment. *Congressional Record.* (Serial No. 15, 1971-10-25). Hearings before Subcommittee No. 3, of the Committee on the Judiciary, House of Representatives, Ninety-Second Congress, *First Session on Corrections, Part II, Prisons, Prison Reform and Prisoner's Rights: California.* Washington, DC: U.S. Government Printing Office.

CHAPTER 9

Client Noncompliance and Termination of Care

CLIENT NONCOMPLIANCE WITH TREATMENT RECOMMENDATIONS

Midwifery is a partnership between a trained professional and a client with a common goal: healthy pregnancy and birth. The relationship is characterized by shared responsibility, which is to say that both the midwife and the client take ownership of behaviors and outcomes. Unlike the medical model, in which patients are relatively passive and expect physicians to be fully responsible for health outcomes, the Midwives Model of Care (MMOC) (Rothman, 1979) posits that clients and midwives collaborate and jointly invest in the quality of the pregnancy and birth. Like any partnership, the cooperative alliance between a midwife and client must strike a balance between the needs of the team and the needs of the individuals. This balance can be upset when a midwife has a practice protocol that the client chooses not to follow.

In many cases, client refusal of a procedure is acceptable and appropriate. For example, when a midwife recommends a newborn screen to parents and informs them of the risks and benefits of the procedure and screening, the midwife rightly places the decision into the hands of the parents. If parents refuse the screen, it behooves the midwife to get the refusal in writing from them, explicitly documenting the midwife's explanation of the risks and benefits of newborn screening.

Documentation of the informed consent process and a written refusal serve dual purposes: to protect the midwife from legal risk in the case of a bad outcome, and to ensure the client has taken full responsibility for knowledgeably refusing a treatment or screening. The National Association of Certified Professional Midwives (NACPM, 2004) instructs its members to clearly document instances when a client's decision conflicts with the midwife's advice as well as instances when a woman's choice is outside the midwife's competency or scope of practice.

Some cases of refusal may place tension on the midwife-client relationship, and may even be grounds for termination of the relationship. For instance, if a midwife deems it necessary for a client to seek medical treatment for a condition that places the woman or her fetus at risk, and the client refuses to do so, the midwife may need to transfer care of the client to an obstetrician who has the skill and capacity to manage the potential complication. Thompson (2007) describes a similar scenario in which a planned home birth becomes a complicated situation that the midwife feels necessitates transfer to a hospital. If the woman refuses to transfer, "the midwife is caught in the ethical (and legal) dilemma of understanding the woman's choice but not agreeing with it" (p. 282). Schorn (2007) states that "when a client refuses treatment that the clinician believes is necessary for the client's health and welfare, ethical principles of beneficence and nonmaleficence can conflict with the principle of patient autonomy" (p. 466).

What are the limits of informed choice, and when does the client, through the denial of recommended treatments, become noncompliant? "The term *noncompliance* is used in medicine particularly in regard to a patient not taking a prescribed medication or following a prescribed course of therapy . . . Noncompliance may be overt (as with a Christian Scientist who rejects recommended therapy for religious reasons) or covert (as with a client who insists she is eating a healthy diet, but her health condition suggests otherwise)" ("Noncompliance," 1999, n.p.).

As the clinician, it is your job to differentiate between situations involving consent and those involving noncompliance. As outlined in Chapter 4, competent adults have the right to autonomy and can refuse treatments. The context of pregnancy complicates informed consent because the fetus experiences the consequences of the actions and inactions of the mother, but this fact does not "strip her of basic rights, or minimize them" (Greenlaw, 1990, p. 156). As midwives, our role in the decision-making process is typically that of an advisor. Yet, if the woman's choice has the potential to result in harm to herself or her fetus, the midwife has an ethical dilemma. Although it is much easier to deal with the autonomous client who chooses what the midwife would advise, clinicians frequently encounter situations in which the client's choices differ from the midwife's preferences. The American College of Nurse-Midwives (ACNM) acknowledges the boundaries of respect: "Respect does not imply automatic agreement with another's decision or actions, nor does it relieve midwives of the obligation to protect others and themselves when choices may cause harm" (2008, p. 3). Therefore, midwives must balance competing ethical demands of client autonomy and nonmaleficence in cases of client noncompliance.

In dealing with issues of noncompliance, direct communication is required to maintain the best interests of the client, the midwife, and the midwife-client relationship. Many healthcare providers fail to effectively communicate with their patients about issues of noncompliance. Sometimes clinicians use coercive techniques (either overt or subtle) to control a patient's behavior. This is a highly unethical abuse of the authority role of the healthcare provider that denies the patient's individual identity and undermines his or her autonomy. Moreover, delivery of a treatment without the client's consent is both unethical and illegal, incurring both civil and criminal liability (Greenlaw, 1990). Respect for autonomy must be maintained when confronting noncompliance, and the best tools for mutual understanding are communicative ones.

Because the well-being of the client is the midwife's primary ethical responsibility, it is a good place to begin a dialogue. This strategy places the conversation within the context of caring. To give your client good care, you must abide by certain protocols. When a client understands that the midwife's perspective is a caring one, defenses are likely to go down, and a genuine exchange of perspectives is more likely.

It is the midwife's responsibility to offer an explanation and even to attempt to persuade a client when the midwife feels that a treatment option is necessary. This is both an ethical and a professional obligation. Beneficence requires a midwife to attempt to demonstrate the essential nature of a treatment to a client when necessary. Further, the midwife is hired to provide a professional opinion and should make her best effort to effectively communicate this to her client.

Practicing active listening techniques enhances communication between a clinician and a client. Perhaps the most valuable communicative tool available, active listening can be studied and honed through practice. It involves attending to the speaker; providing cues that you are attending, such as nods or verbal affirmations (e.g., "yes," "I see," "okay"); and reflecting the meaning of the speaker's words through paraphrase or repeating the speaker's words verbatim, without added judgment. An active listener waits for feedback from the speaker indicating that the reflected meanings are correct or need clarification. When a client is attended to in this manner, she is likely to express herself fully. For more information on how to learn to be an active listener, see Ivey, Ivey, and Zalaquett (2009). One of the most important skills to being a good clinician is to listen to your clients. Midwives who practice active listening are demonstrating caring and respect for clients by attending to their clients' words, mirroring and reflecting them with appropriate gestures and verbal responses.

Ensuring the client's full comprehension of the situation is vital to effective communication. Depending on the client and the nature of the conflict, additional supportive elements, such as a reference article or the attendance of the client's spouse or a mediator, may be required. The goal is not to overwhelm a client with your evidence or justify your stance; rather, it is to effectively explain and support your position in a manner that is meaningful to that client. For some clients, a peer-reviewed journal article is valued. Others may prefer information in the form of personal anecdotes and case studies. The presence of a third party who can bridge the gap of understanding between clinician and client may be pivotal to effective communication between parties, especially when there is dissonance. For example, if a client is using drugs despite the midwife's warnings, the midwife may request that the client's partner meet with them to be informed of the risks of drug use in pregnancy. The presence of the partner may help facilitate clear communication between the midwife and client, and may be helpful if termination of care is sought by either party.

Dealing with noncompliance may be a boundary issue for the midwife. In situations of noncompliance where risk is incurred by both client and midwife, the midwife must act in accordance with the client's best interest. Yet, the midwife is justified in taking action to protect herself and her practice from harm. In these cases, and many others, collaboration, referral, or termination of care may be appropriate.

TERMINATION OF CARE

"The partnership between a woman and a midwife may be ended by either party" (ACNM, 2008, p. 6). When a client decides to terminate care with a midwife, the midwife is not completely free of obligation to the client until the client has established care with another provider. The ethical logistics related to a client's decision to terminate care are less complicated than when a midwife decides to terminate the clinical relationship.

Termination of the midwifery relationship is a very serious matter. The woman has hired the midwife with the expectation of continuity of care through her postpartum period, typically. Issues of fidelity must be considered when a midwife terminates care. However, there are appropriate situations in which to terminate care with a client, and we explore most of these and the inherent risks involved. Ethical guidelines for practitioners for handling termination of care are provided.

The most common reason for termination is scope of practice or competency. When a client develops a complication that is outside the midwife's skill set, it is imperative that the midwife transfer care to a physician if collaboration or referral will not adequately meet the client's needs. For example, placenta previa requires a surgical delivery and presents risk to the pregnancy. Hence, transfer of care to a physician during pregnancy is imperative for the well-being of both mother and fetus. Aside from an obstetrical complication, midwives may terminate care for a number of reasons.

NACPM grants its members the right to refuse care in situations that are either unsafe or unacceptable, and further states that the midwife has a *respon-*

sibility to transfer care when necessary for safety (2004). Placenta previa is unsafe, so a midwife has an obligation to transfer care. An unacceptable situation may be anything from client noncompliance to a dangerous or threatening situation for the midwife. Other professions have also addressed termination issues in their professional documents. For example, "Psychologists may terminate therapy when threatened or otherwise endangered by the client/patient or another person with whom the client/patient has a relationship" (American Psychological Association, 2002, p. 16). Similarly, "counselors may terminate counseling when in jeopardy of harm by the client, or another person with whom the client has a relationship, or when clients do not pay fees as agreed upon" (American Counseling Association, 2005, p. 6). There is no clear guideline for midwives on the ethics of termination of care on the basis of nonpayment. Anne Frye (1998) offers some suggestions on negotiating with clients regarding issues of nonpayment that work toward maintaining the relationship. These include clear communication regarding payment and refunds, maintaining accurate financial records, and payment in advance.

A study published in the *Journal of Midwifery and Women's Health* (Schorn, 2007) found that termination of care was rare, and that there are a myriad of reasons that midwives make the decision to end the midwife-client relationship. Of the 111 study participants, the average midwife discharged 1.36 clients during her career. Noncompliance, obnoxious or abusive behavior, and failure to keep appointments were the most frequently cited reasons for discharge from midwifery care. Comments from midwives provided greater insight into the dynamics involved when midwives discharge clients. Drug-seeking behavior and lack of therapeutic partnership were reported as additional grounds for discharge. The author emphasizes the essential roles of effective communication and mutual respect for resolving conflicts in the midwife-client relationship.

Perhaps the most important aspect of termination of care is the midwife-client relationship. Once a clinical relationship has been established, midwives have a responsibility of nonmaleficence to the client. The ethical principle of fidelity underlies the midwife's relational obligation to the client. The client's ability to trust and her social or emotional stability may be at risk. Pregnancy may present further psychological vulnerabilities that may intensify the woman's reaction to being rejected by her midwife. Therefore, a decision to terminate should be considered carefully. Weighing the risks and benefits of termination will give the midwife insights into the decision to terminate care.

The care of the client may be put at risk by terminating care because changing providers disrupts continuity. The midwife will have knowledge of the woman and her pregnancy, some of which is not relevant to the client's chart. Again, the ethical principle of nonmaleficence is involved. The midwife must not do harm to the client by termination of care. At the very least, the midwife has an obligation to ensure that another appropriate care provider is in place. Even under the best circumstances, the client will have to start over in developing a relationship with a provider for her pregnancy and birth.

Because of the inherent risks involved, termination should only be sought when no other viable solution exists. When it is appropriate for the midwife to terminate the relationship, specific steps are required to protect the client from harm. These involve communication, avoidance of both a gap in care and abandonment, and proper documentation.

Communication is the midwife's most important tool. Midwives have a responsibility to clearly communicate with the client about a decision to terminate care. The client's dignity and autonomy are involved in such a decision, as well as the midwife's duty of fidelity. In maintaining the client's dignity, good communication is essential. The woman needs to be included in, or at least adequately informed of, the process. Termination of care tests the boundaries of autonomy. An autonomous person may or may not choose to end the relationship with her midwife. When the midwife decides to terminate, it is usually because she has very clear reasons for doing so that protect the midwife's own autonomy. The client must either accept the midwife's decision or make grievances against the decision. To uphold the principle of fidelity, the midwife should put her own personal needs aside for the client's best interest (Beauchamp & Childress, 2009). As a rule, midwives must reflect on their own biases and act according to the client's best interest during a termination of care. Termination situations can be complex and difficult to judge. The midwife may seek consultation from a peer to assist her in clarifying her priorities prior to proceeding with a termination.

Once a decision has been made to transfer care, the midwife must take great care to minimize risk to her client. Great harm could come to a client if the midwife failed to provide a seamless transfer of care. The client could go weeks or months without prenatal care while in search of a new care provider. A gap in care must be avoided. Midwives are required to continue to provide care until the transfer is complete (NACPM, 2004). The International Confederation of Midwives (ICM) further requires a midwife to "refuse to provide care only if someone else is available to provide the needed care" (2003, p. 3). The availability of another care provider may be difficult to define, especially in rural areas. Some families may choose an unassisted birth over hospital-based care if another midwife is unavailable. Yet, if a competent maternity provider accepts a referral, the midwife is not responsible for the decisions that parents make once the referral has been made. Providing appropriate referrals is the midwife's responsibility. The new care provider should be someone who is qualified to care for the specific needs of the client. Ensuring that the client has a new provider in place goes a long way toward preventing abandonment.

Definitions of abandonment in clinical care vary across disciplines. From a general biomedical ethics perspective, abandonment of a patient is a breach of fidelity (Beauchamp & Childress, 2009). For example, a midwife deciding to end a clinical relationship without the consent of the client represents a failure to live up to one's obligation or duty. A midwife practicing in an out-of-hospital setting must accompany a client when transport during labor is necessary; to do otherwise is abandonment. From a psychotherapeutic perspective, discussion of abandonment focuses on the emotional experiences of loss and abandonment. In the medical field, abandonment is more narrowly defined in terms of ending care of a patient without providing appropriate transfer of care (American Medical Association, 2006). From a judicial perspective, "abandonment is a legal term which refers to the wrongful cessation of the provision of care" (Schorn, 2007, p. 466). A definition provided by Schorn more specifically for midwives notes that abandonment must initially include established fidelity, followed by breach of duty and subsequent injury. Injury may occur when a provider discontinues care with a client without providing for appropriate referral such that quality care can be continued. Legal and ethical issues are separate. Although one may legally discharge a client, ethical considerations should be prioritized.

A midwife must take all measures possible to prevent abandonment and properly document the discharge of a client. Establishing written guidelines for discharging clients and following those guidelines is advisable. While taking steps to consciously avoid abandonment and a gap in care, the midwife must document each step involved in the termination of a clinical relationship. When a client's termination is based on noncompliance, for example, the midwife must chart the specific behaviors that constitute noncompliance. When the midwife communicates to the client about termination of care, this too must be documented. All actions taken in providing referral, such as faxing records and communication with other professionals, must be charted accurately. The process of documentation of a transfer of care is beneficent. Midwives make every effort to accurately document all aspects of care for the benefit of the client.

The professionalism of midwives in handling a termination reflects on midwives' care for their clients. Midwives approach their work from a caring perspective in the service of women and their families. If a midwife denies the client clear communication, fails to provide appropriate referral, allows a gap in care, or abandons a client, her actions reflect poorly on the profession. Sometimes a midwife's own needs conflict with that of her client, but fidelity requires the midwife to prioritize the client's needs. Still, there may be times when a midwife has to maintain boundaries in order to protect herself, her client, or her practice from harm. These situations can be very difficult to manage ethically. When in doubt, seek consultation with colleagues. Consider what actions would best reflect the MMOC and uphold dignity, autonomy, and fidelity.

CASE EXAMPLES

CASE 1

Amie is a southern rural midwife working with an underserved population. Her client, Teresa, has positive glucosuria at two consecutive prenatal appointments. Amie counsels Teresa about nutrition, and requests that she maintain a food journal to bring to the next prenatal exam. Teresa does not comply with the midwife's request, and has glucosuria for a third time on the morning of her 28-week glucose screen. Her fasting glucose level is 100 mg/dL, and a two-hour glucose screen is 140 mg/dL. Because of the results of the fasting and postprandial screens, Amie's protocols guide her to follow up with a glucose tolerance test. This test also comes in borderline.

In Amie's experience, women benefit from nutritional counseling after borderline glucose screen results, and subsequent tests are usually in range. If the blood glucose level can be controlled with diet, the client remains low risk and can continue with midwifery care if random glucose tests stay in the normal range. If diet has no effect on the results and random glucose screens are out of range, the midwife needs to transfer client care to a physician.

Amie discusses the results of the test with Teresa, going into detail about the risks of gestational diabetes. She further explains that a woman who has this disorder requires physician care. Amie tells Teresa that she can remain in midwifery care as long as she maintains normal blood glucose levels. Amie emphasizes the importance of a low-sugar, high-protein diet and a variety of whole grains and vegetables. Again, she requests that Teresa maintain a food journal.

At the next appointment, two weeks later, Teresa has positive glucosuria. A random glucose screen shows her blood glucose level at 138 mg/dL. Teresa doesn't have the diet journal and is defensive with Amie when questioned about her food intake.

Questions

1. Is Teresa being noncompliant?
2. What tools does Amie have for handling this situation?
3. How are boundaries involved in this case?

Analysis

The best tool for working with a client who is challenging boundaries is communication. The midwife must strive to improve communication with this client. A good place to begin is through active listening. When Teresa becomes agitated or resistant about nutritional counseling, Amie has the opportunity to explore her client's reaction. For example, Amie might ask, "Do you feel uncomfortable with nutritional counseling?" or "I notice that when we discuss your diet, the tone of our conversation becomes tense." Directly addressing the client's resistance to nutritional therapy is a good place to begin a conversation about noncompliance.

Perhaps the client is not being noncompliant. Rather, she may be indirectly refusing a treatment. The midwife, Amie, will not be able to differentiate between a consent issue and a noncompliance issue unless she asks. She can ask follow-up questions, such as "Do you want nutritional counseling for this problem?" If the client refuses nutritional counseling, the midwife can then move forward with her care. She may chart the client's refusal and refer to her protocols regarding gestational diabetes screens, while discussing blood glucose levels that define gestational diabetes with the client and explaining the requirement to transfer care to a physician if appropriate.

While working with this client, Amie must protect her professional boundaries. She can simultaneously best serve the needs of her client and work within her practice protocols if she is clear with herself and her client about her scope of practice and the risks of gestational diabetes. Through improved communication, Amie and Teresa can navigate their relationship and determine an appropriate plan of care.

CASE 2

Darleen begins care with Ruth for her first pregnancy at 20 weeks. It becomes clear to Ruth at the initial appointment that Darleen and her partner are struggling financially. Darleen has a part-time job in the service industry, and her partner, Randy, is a student. Ruth's practice does not accept Medicaid, but the care is affordable compared to a physician's. Ruth advises the couple to apply for Medicaid, but explains that her fees must be privately paid.

The couple chooses an affordable payment plan for their midwifery care. Yet, it is clear after a few months that the couple is not able to make their payments. The midwifery practice has a clearly written financial agreement that requires timely payment for services rendered. Because the midwifery practice has no financial department, when Darleen doesn't make her payments, Ruth must address this with her directly.

Questions

1. What are Ruth's responsibilities to Darleen and her partner?
2. How do financial boundaries factor into quality client care?

3. How should midwives structure their practices to meet the needs of low-income women and their families?
4. Does the midwife have a basis for termination of care?

Analysis

Financial compensation for midwifery care has been the subject of analysis. The right to fair compensation for services rendered is a largely agreed-upon principle in midwifery (Association of Texas Midwives, 2009; Frye, 1998). Compensation may vary depending on region, experience (ACNM, 2004), and practice setting (Brucker, 2004). When a midwife works for a larger institution or organization, it may be unnecessary for her to communicate with clients about payment. Because many midwives earn salaries from an employer, their pay is not dependent on a particular client's payment arrangements. In these cases, it is unlikely that payment boundaries will have a bearing on client care.

Alternatively, when midwives work in private practice, they have more intimate knowledge of client payment arrangements and may be financially dependent on clients making payments in a timely manner. When clients fail to meet their financial obligations to the midwife, the clinical relationship may be at risk. Working with women who are of limited financial means may create challenges to fair compensation for midwifery care. (Please see Chapter 6 for more information about maintaining financial boundaries with clients.)

Once Ruth accepts a client into her practice, she has an ethical obligation to provide quality care to this client and maintain the client's best interests. However, the client also has an ethical obligation to pay for midwifery care. When the client does not pay for services rendered, the clinical relationship may be put at risk. This can impair the care that the client receives.

The midwife must clearly communicate financial policies with clients prior to rendering services. A financial contract is an appropriate means of doing so, but discussing the matter verbally can help clear up any misconceptions. Once a midwife enters the clinical relationship with the client, it is more difficult to negotiate financial matters. The focus of the midwife-client relationship should not be financial, but clinical.

Because Darleen entered a financial agreement with Ruth, she is obligated to render payment according to the terms of the agreement. If she does not do so, and the consequences of failure to pay are clearly outlined in the agreement, then the midwife may choose to stick to the agreement. Alternatively, the midwife may renegotiate and discuss optional payment plans with the client. The final alternative for Ruth is to provide care regardless of payment. If the midwife is willing to work without payment for services, she must provide the same quality of care that she would if the client were paying.

If the contract clearly states that termination may result from failure to meet the terms of financial agreement, then there is a legal basis for termination of care. Is this ethical? Termination of care is a serious action that midwives rarely take. If the midwife continues to provide care until the transfer of care to an appropriate provider is complete, then she has met her ethical obligations in the relationship. Still, the question remains whether a monetary barrier to health care is ethical.

The ethical principle of justice factors into issues related to socioeconomic barriers in health care. Some of the ethical codes address the midwife's responsibility to provide care to all women, regardless of socioeconomic status (ACNM, 2008; Midwives Alliance of North America, 1997). One must not discriminate against a client on the basis of her financial state. Although midwives are not obligated to work for free, they may refer women and their families to Medicaid and assist low-income women in finding alternative methods of payment. Midwives have options for supporting justice in health care. On an individual level, a practitioner may choose to take a low-income client pro bono, for example. On a local, state, or national level, midwives can organize support for programs or bills that support healthcare reform and make midwifery care accessible for all.

CASE 3

Dalia hires her midwife, Abby, after interviewing several midwives. She identifies with Abby's intellectualism and evidence-based practice guidelines. Dalia desires continuity of care throughout her pregnancy and birth, and Abby agrees to these terms. She sees clients at her office adjacent to the hospital, and usually takes three call shifts per week. However, Abby agrees to be on-call for specific clients on an individual basis.

When Dalia is 32 weeks along in her pregnancy, Abby informs her that there is a conference in another city that is scheduled near the time of her birth. Abby has made plans to attend the conference, and may miss Dalia's birth should it conflict with the conference. Dalia is visibly upset, and accuses Abby of breaking her word. Abby listens to Dalia, affirms her feelings, but insists that she's committed to attending the conference and will not change her plans. Dalia fires her on the spot.

Questions

1. What responsibilities does Abby owe this client?
2. When is it acceptable for a midwife to break an agreement with a client?

3. What factors might Abby consider in making a decision whether or not to attend the conference?

Analysis

When midwives make verbal agreements with clients to attend their births, the midwife should make every effort to uphold those agreements. Of course, the nature of our work may sometimes prevent our availability at every birth. Two clients may labor simultaneously at different locations, for example. Midwives should be open and honest about their availability and provide clients information about alternative arrangements for care when the midwife is unavailable.

Abby made a clear commitment to attend Dalia's birth. Dalia's decision to hire Abby may have been made on the basis of this commitment. By breaking this agreement with Dalia, Abby undermined the client's trust. This could be considered a breach of ethics, in that it caused the client harm. However, because Abby is an autonomous human being, she also has a right to make decisions that are in her best interest. Perhaps she had a rare opportunity to present at the conference. To forego this opportunity may seem unthinkable to Abby, who values research and intellectual inquiry. The unilateral decision that Abby made to break an agreement with a client was clearly not in the client's best interest. By putting her own needs before the client's, Abby is guilty of infidelity.

Is it ever acceptable for a midwife to make a decision that serves her own needs over those of her client? This question may be analyzed from a number of perspectives. One could argue that what is best for the midwife is best for the client. If Abby made a huge contribution to the field of midwifery by presenting valuable information at the conference, then it might be argued that her client indirectly benefits from Abby's decision to attend the conference. However, the client's immediate needs are the most relevant to the midwife-client relationship. There may be situations in which the midwife's own needs may be put before those of the client, especially in situations where the benefit of serving one's own needs far outweighs the benefit of serving the client's. Consider a situation in which a midwife's child is ill. The midwife is also a mother, and her role of caring for and comforting her child may be more important than her role of providing routine prenatal care, which the client needs, but which can be delayed.

If Abby felt torn between her commitment to her client and her commitment to research, she might have chosen to discuss the conflict with Dalia. If Dalia had had an opportunity to give input regarding Abby's decision, perhaps she would have felt differently about Abby's conflict. If Abby had explained that she was only going to be away for a day or two, Dalia could consider the risks and benefits of Abby's departure.

Abby has a responsibility to Dalia to protect her from harm, to provide quality care, to uphold her dignity and autonomy, and to prioritize her needs. Even though Dalia fired her, Abby still has these responsibilities, along with the additional responsibility to provide an appropriate referral for Dalia. She will need to maintain care of this client until another care provider has taken over fully.

REFERENCES

American College of Nurse-Midwives (ACNM). (2004). *Select results of ACNM compensation & benefits survey.* Retrieved August 9, 2009, from http://www.midwife.org/siteFiles/education/ACNM_salary_survey_2005.pdf

American College of Nurse-Midwives (ACNM). (2008). *American College of Nurse-Midwives code of ethics with explanatory statements.* Silver Spring, MD: Author.

American Counseling Association. (2005). *Code of ethics.* Retrieved July 7, 2009, from http://www.counseling.org/Resources/CodeOfEthics/TP/Home/CT2.aspx

American Medical Association (AMA). (2006). *Code of medical ethics.* Retrieved August 9, 2009, from http://www.ama-assn.org/ama/pub/physician-resources/medical-ethics/code-medical-ethics.shtml

American Psychological Association (APA). (2002). *Ethical principles of psychologists and code of conduct.* Retrieved August 9, 2009, from http://www.apa.org/ethics/code2002.pdf

Association of Texas Midwives. (2009). *Code for ethical midwifery practice.* Retrieved August 9, 2009, from http://www.texasmidwives.com/code.asp

Beauchamp, T. L., & Childress, J. F. (2009). *Principles of biomedical ethics* (6th ed.). New York: Oxford University Press.

Brucker, M. C. (2004). *What compensation arrangements should a nurse midwife consider when starting a practice?* Retrieved October 15, 2009, from http://www.medscape.com/viewarticle/471339

Frye, A. (1998). *Holistic midwifery: A comprehensive textbook for midwives in homebirth practice: Vol. 1. Care during pregnancy.* Portland, OR: Labrys Press.

Greenlaw, J. L. (1990). Treatment refusal, noncompliance, and substance abuse in pregnancy: Legal and ethical issues. *Birth, 17*(3), 152–156.

International Confederation of Midwives (ICM). (2003). *ICM international code of ethics for midwives.* Retrieved January 30, 2009, from http://www.internationalmidwives.org/Documentation/Coredocuments/tabid/322/Default.aspx

Ivey, A. E., Ivey, M. B., & Zalaquett, C. P. (2009). *Intentional interviewing and counseling: Facilitating client development in a multicultural society.* Belmont, CA: Brooks/Cole.

Midwives Alliance of North America (MANA). (1997). *Statement of values and ethics.* Washington, DC: Author.

National Association of Certified Professional Midwives (NACPM). (2004). *Essential documents of the National Association of Certified Professional Midwives.* Retrieved August 9, 2009, from http://www.nacpm.org/Resources/nacpm-standards.pdf

Noncompliance. (1999). Retrieved August 9, 2009, from http://www.medterms.com/script/main/art.asp?articlekey=10159

Rothman, B. K. (1979). *Two models in maternity care: Defining and negotiating reality.* New York: New York University Press.

Schorn, M. N. (2007). Midwives' practices and beliefs about discharging clients from their practice. *Journal of Midwifery and Women's Health, 52*(5), 465–472.

Thompson, J. E. (2007). Professional ethics. In L. A. Ament (Ed.), *Professional issues in midwifery.* Sudbury, MA: Jones and Bartlett.

CHAPTER 10

Diversity, Equity, and Justice

Most clinical and helping professions have established standards of care and ethical behavior. As we have discussed in previous chapters, such standards serve multiple purposes and the interests of both the public and members of the profession. More recently, society has placed an increased emphasis on the need to incorporate notions of diversity, equity, and justice in published guidelines for healthcare providers (Carr & DeJoseph, 2001). The goal of this chapter is to identify key concepts related to the ethics of diversity and justice such that midwives have access to resources that facilitate just and equitable interactions with others.

A review of the ethical codes in midwifery indicates that the notion of justice has already been incorporated in some of our professional organizations' views of ethical practice. For example, the preamble of the code of the International Confederation of Midwives (ICM) states, "This code acknowledges women as persons with human rights, seeks justice for all people and equity in access to health care, and is based on mutual relationships of respect, trust, and the dignity of all members of society" (2003, p. 1; see Appendix D). The code of the American College of Nurse-Midwives (ACNM) notes that "the call for all midwives to respect their own self worth and dignity stems from the same ethical principles, respect for autonomy, and justice, that require midwives to honor the human rights and the dignity of all people" (2008, p. 4; see Appendix C). Similarly, the code of the Nursing and Midwifery Council requires that midwives "demonstrate a personal and professional commitment to equality and diversity" (2008, p. 5; see Appendix F). Consequently, we must explore the concepts of justice, diversity, and equity so that we may better apply these constructs to the daily practice of midwifery.

It should come as no surprise that midwives are aware of and sensitive to issues of diversity and justice, as we work with a diverse public. The stereotypical nuclear family (think *Leave It to Beaver*) represents fewer than 10% of American households. As technology permits older women to reproduce and the age of menarche is lower, the age at which women can give birth has been extended significantly. Moreover, families are now self-defined rather than externally defined (i.e., a family is defined not as a married couple with children, but rather by the individuals who live together, such as two women and their baby) (Carr & DeJoseph, 2001). Diversity is not merely an idea; diversity is a key component of daily practice.

SOME CONCEPTUAL AND PRACTICAL CHALLENGES

Concepts of justice, diversity, and equity lack some of the concreteness that other ethical ideas carry. Consequently, the day-to-day application of these constructs in the work of midwives may be less apparent than that of consent and confidentiality. Williamson and Harrison (2001) note that "there is surprisingly little consensus about the meaning of terms such as cultural sensitivity and cultural appropriate care. Nor are there reflections on incorporating these concepts into practice" (p. 22). Without a clear, shared meaning of these abstract yet important concepts, midwives may struggle to find guidance in providing just, compassionate, and equitable care to diverse client populations.

In an effort to overcome conceptual barriers, we offer some basic definitions of key concepts related to justice and diversity. We agree with Williamson and Harrison's (2001) assertion that "there is little clarity about definitions or about how these amorphous concepts might be incorporated into practice" (p. 22). Nevertheless, we strive for greater clarity by referencing definitions that we find useful as a starting point toward reaching the goal of culturally competent practice in midwifery.

Before we offer some definitions of terms to mitigate conceptual barriers, we must first acknowledge a practical obstacle between current and more just practices. Historically, the wealthy and powerful (e.g., the American Medical Association) have been the most influential in developing and influencing healthcare policy, while marginalized groups (e.g., midwifery organizations) have been left without much of a voice in the process (Harrod, Hanson, & Osborne, 2007). Although there have been significant moves toward better political organizing among midwives (e.g., the Midwives Political Action Committee, Midwives and Mothers in Action), midwives must continually work to ensure that their voices and the voices of those they serve are part of the health policy discussion.

We also recognize that access to midwifery services may be limited by a number of factors. The legal status of midwifery varies across states and is often under attack, and women who qualify for Medicaid have learned that some states do not provide Medicaid coverage for midwifery services. A healthcare system that denies low-income women access to quality maternity care from midwives (often at a lower cost than physician care) raises serious questions about justice and equity for all women and babies. Just as there is a documented "achievement gap" in education between whites and minorities, so too a healthcare gap exists and is widening (Boufford & Lee, 2002). As we write this book in the midst of a national discourse on healthcare reform, we are mindful of the need to develop policies that serve everyone.

There are also points at which the conceptual and practical intersect. For example, utilitarian ethical theory (conceptual) has direct implications for the distribution of limited healthcare resources (practical). Utilitarianism is often explained as "the greatest good for the greatest number of people," which is to say that decisions are made based on a quantitative approach. Hinman (2008) provides hypothetical cases that challenge our ideas of what is right and just. For example, you are the chief of police in a small community that has been terrorized by violent crimes. The perpetrator has died in an accident, but you are unable to persuade the public that he was responsible for the crimes. You have arrested a transient and could frame him for the crimes, putting the public at ease. From a utilitarian perspective, the conviction of the transient under false pretense would result in the greatest happiness, because the townspeople would feel safe and secure. Some might call this "doing the wrong thing for the right reasons," but it has also led others to reject utilitarianism.

In writing about ethical philosophies in the context of midwifery practice, Jones (2000) finds fault with utilitarianism, noting that it "can place unreasonable demands on individuals, considering everyone as equal when clearly they are often unequal" (p. 18). If one believes that people are interchangeable and can be reduced to quantities, then utilitarianism has fewer limitations. But if one holds that there are real and tangible differences, that individuals have unique characteristics, and that cultural and societal forces yield inequalities, then utilitarianism becomes problematic. For example, women with children have different responsibilities than women without children, so some would argue that they should not be treated as equals when policy decisions are made (Jones, 2000).

The concept of *justice* has a long and rich history in the world of ideas. Exploring the nuances of justice reminds us that what appears to be a simple and straightforward term challenges our preconceived notions. Hinman (2008) offers two definitions: *distributive justice* refers to "a theory about how best to allocate the benefits and burdens of society among individuals," whereas *retributive justice* refers to "a theory about how best to respond to injustice in society" (p. 365). When lawmakers decide whether midwifery care will be covered by finite healthcare dollars, their decisions concern distributive justice. When a healthcare practitioner is sued for malpractice, the court's procedures revolve around retributive justice. Additionally, Young (1990) addresses justice as a means of confronting discrimination and oppression. For example, discrimination against individuals because of their ethnicity, sexual orientation, or sex is incompatible with a just society.

In Western culture, the idea of justice dates back to Plato. In *The Republic*, various notions of justice are discussed and ultimately rejected, leading up to Plato's view of justice as

> harmony, both internal and external. Internal harmony is a proper balance in the soul, and external harmony manifests itself in the state. The virtuous individual must live in a just society. Thus, inner and outer justice need one another: Without just individuals, a just society is impossible; without a just society, the life of the just individual may not be a happy one. (Hinman, 2008, p. 236)

John Rawls was perhaps the most influential modern contributor to our understanding of justice. In Rawls's seminal work, *A Theory of Justice* (1971), he focuses on egalitarianism, reflecting his passion for the fair treatment of all persons. In his model of distributive justice, Rawls argues that when one is put in the position of representing others for the purposes of defining the policies that will distribute resources and govern society, one must be behind a hypothetical "veil of ignorance." Behind the veil of ignorance, one knows nothing about those for whom one is making decisions. Their sex, race, socioeconomic status, and other characteristics remain invisible. Consequently, one's decisions should be egalitarian because they are not based on stereotypes or prejudice. In this respect, fairness is defined by treating everyone as equals.

Critics of Rawls's approach argue that the veil of ignorance is not useful for practical, day-to-day decision making because we do not in fact live behind a veil of ignorance. We are very much aware of race, sex, ability, and many other individual differences that often influence how we interact with and treat one another. Other critics note that individual differences are real and in some cases should be taken into account when making decisions about the distribution of resources. For example, some advocates of affirmative action believe that resources should not be equally distributed in a society that has historically been unequal. Similarly, accommodations are made for people with disabilities in recognition of their differences.

Recall from Chapter 1 that justice is one of the broad ethical principles of common morality that serve as a framework for biomedical ethical thought (Beauchamp & Childress, 2009). Midwives have an ethical obligation to treat clients, colleagues, and other collaborators justly, which is to say that respect, fairness, and egalitarianism should guide our interactions with others.

We will return to the concept of justice as applied to midwifery care, but first must establish a shared understanding of some critical terms that we use in this chapter: *culture, race, ethnicity, sex, gender,* and *sexual orientation.* Following these definitions, we will proceed with a model of culturally competent midwifery practice and some case examples.

- *Culture:* Culture refers to "a pattern of learned behaviors, attitudes, beliefs, and values exhibited by a group that shares a common history and usually geographic proximity" (Carr & DeJoseph, 2001, p. 211). Culture may be independent of race or ethnicity (defined below) and is best conceptualized as shared beliefs and values. Signs of cultural definers have been observed in groups as varied as competitive barbershop quartet singers, homeschoolers, "Trekkies" (avid fans of *Star Trek*), and knitters. One could even argue that there is a culture of midwifery. The term is complicated because it often overlaps with other categories, such as religion (consider Jewish culture as an example).

- *Race:* Race may be one of the most complex and politically charged terms used to define individuals and groups. Historically, race has been conceptualized based on physical characteristics and assumptions about genetics. The term, as Carr and DeJoseph (2001) note, is "by no means biologically useful" (p. 211). Nevertheless, the concept of race is significant both politically and socially. The way we use the concept of race validates the notion of the political taking precedence over the biological. For example, the child of a Caucasian mother and African American father will be regarded as African American (e.g., Barack Obama is hailed as the first African American president of the United States).

- *Ethnicity:* Similar to the concept of culture, *ethnicity* refers to a group of people "who share cultural, social, and political ties . . . [and] may also share language, history, religion, economic interdependence, and a set of social values" (Carr & DeJoseph, 2001, p. 211). One's ethnic identity may, in some cases, be more salient than other affiliations (e.g., a Korean American's ethnicity may play a more significant role in her identity than her participation in ballroom dancing culture). Often, when individuals use the term *race*, it would be more accurate if they used the term *ethnicity* instead.

- *Sex and gender:* Although the terms *sex* and *gender* have distinct meanings, many use the terms interchangeably, creating much confusion about these important identifiers. The biological status of being male or female (as defined by chromosomes, reproductive organs, etc.) marks one's sex. For example, Jennifer's sex is female (e.g., she has ovaries, a uterus, and a vagina; her 23rd pair of chromosomes is XX). *Gender* refers to the traits that culture ascribes to the biological sexes: "she is feminine" or "she is masculine." Biological males and females may have both feminine and masculine attributes. *Androgyny* refers to having both traditionally masculine and feminine traits and is regarded by some as healthy and balanced.

- *Sexual orientation:* Most people report that they are romantically and sexually attracted to members of the opposite (we prefer the term "other") sex and have a *heterosexual* orientation. A substantial minority of the population reports romantic and sexual attraction to members of the same sex and have a *homosexual* orientation. Others report that they are attracted to men and women and have a *bisexual* orientation. Women who are attracted to women are often referred to as *lesbians*, and men who are attracted to men are often referred to as *gay* (Table 10-1). Note that one's orientation may be invisible and unrelated to behaviors. For example, a woman who is attracted to other women may marry a man for complex reasons (social, economic, reproductive, etc.). How one feels and how one behaves do not necessarily match up, and self-identification or labeling may not conform to established terms (e.g., a woman might call herself "queer" rather than "lesbian"; some people engage in same-sex behaviors but do not self-identify as homosexual or bisexual).

Many employers and institutions have nondiscrimination policies that list various categories like the ones we have just defined. For example, a private school states that it does not discriminate on the basis of "race, color, religion, national origin or disability." These lists are problematic in that they may be interpreted to mean that discrimination against groups who are not listed is assumed to be acceptable. Consider a more inclusive list in the American Psychological Association's code of ethics (2002):

> Psychologists are aware of and respect cultural, individual, and role differences, including those based on age, gender, gender identity, race, ethnicity, culture, national origin, religion, sexual orientation, disability, language, and socioeconomic status and consider these factors when working with members of such groups. (p. 4)

Sexual orientation is mentioned in the ethics codes of both the Midwives Alliance of North American (MANA, 1997) and the American College of Nurse-Midwives (2008). The MANA code states, "We value caring for women to the

---

Table 10-1   Sex, Attraction, and Sexual Orientation

	Biological Female	**Biological Male**
Attracted to men	Heterosexual	Homosexual (gay)
Attracted to women	Homosexual (lesbian)	Heterosexual
Attracted to men and women	Bisexual	Bisexual

best of our ability without prejudice against their age, race, religion, culture, sexual orientation, physical abilities or socioeconomic background" (p. 4). The ACNM code includes the following statement: "Midwives in all aspects of their own professional practice will . . . act without discrimination based on factors such as age, gender, race, ethnicity, religion, lifestyle, sexual orientation, socioeconomic status, disability, or nature of the health problem" (p. 8). These are the only codes that specifically reference sexual orientation.

Having a working knowledge of these key terms helps midwives communicate about difference and diversity by establishing a common language or shared vocabulary regarding some of the salient cultural definers that are frequently encountered in midwifery practice. We recognize that there are other significant categories in addition to the terms defined earlier. Social class, age, religion, political affiliation, and marital status, among other characteristics, are relevant in maternity care. These characteristics often influence our interactions with others. Therefore, we must be cognizant of their potential impact on our relationships and make a conscious effort to prevent prejudice and discrimination. We now shift our focus to the overarching concept of *cultural competence* in midwifery as an ethical concern.

CULTURAL COMPETENCE

The idea of cultural competence in health care and mental health has emerged and evolved over the past decade. Although there is some consensus that midwives and other care providers should develop cultural competence, the field has yet to establish clearly defined objectives for learning such skills. Midwives must be aware that they serve diverse populations. Kennedy, Erickson-Owens, and Davis (2006) reported survey data collected from members of the American College of Nurse-Midwives indicating that although most ACNM members sampled were white females (88.8%), the clients they served were significantly more diverse (only 58.4% white). Note that these "demographic characteristics" are limited to sex and race/ethnicity and do not account for other important aspects of diversity. Nevertheless, the need for some form of cultural competence among midwives is apparent.

Cultural competence has been framed as acknowledging and respecting cultural differences while simultaneously working to minimize negative consequences associated with these differences (Paasche-Orlow, 2004). Although the term *cultural competence* has established itself in the literature, we want to emphasize that the objective of developing such competence must extend *beyond* culture to other differences described earlier (e.g., age, ethnicity, sexual orientation). Therefore, "cultural competence" is a bit of a misnomer. Although "diversity competence" may be a more accurate term, we defer to the convention of using the former term, but our intention is to use it in the broadest sense.

Why is cultural competence an ethical concern? Very little has been written on this topic. Although medicine has a substantial body of literature on the subject of cultural competence, the relationship between ethics and cultural competence is absent (Paasche-Orlow, 2004). Here we provide an introduction to the ethics of cultural competence. Acknowledging, respecting, appreciating, and tolerating differences relate directly to the ethical principle of justice, particularly in the context of Young's (1990) conceptualization of justice as a means of eliminating oppression and discrimination. Moreover, understanding and working with difference results in better care (recall *beneficence*), and failure to recognize and understand significant cultural factors can result in harm (recall *nonmaleficence*).

Paasche-Orlow (2004) argues that although culturally competent care is often promoted for utilitarian reasons (e.g., to improve the quality of care), on a more fundamental level it is an extension of both justice and autonomy. "The ethics of cultural competence involves (1) learning about culture, (2) the embrace of pluralism, and (3) accommodation" (Paasche-Orlow, 2004, p. 350). Learning about other cultures is an admirable starting point and much can be gained from a beginning anthropology or sociology course. However, mere knowledge of other cultures is insufficient for ethical practice; one must also embrace pluralism and make efforts to accommodate. Pluralism is a value system that holds that there are diverse views, beliefs, and perspectives and that we should not assume that everyone shares our values, beliefs, and perspectives (nor should we impose ours on others). Moreover, pluralism discourages judgment based on differences. One further step in ethical cultural competence involves the clinician exercising accommodation rather than placing this expectation on clients. When accommodating, a midwife does not expect the client to adapt to her cultural practices but meets the client where she is. This does not require the midwife to adapt her own personal set of values. In fact, setting a tone of acceptance for diversity can be accomplished through honest discourse about differences.

The term *cultural humility* (Tervalon & Murray-García, 1998) has been proposed as an alternative to cultural competence. Those critical of cultural competence argue that it is assessed at a surface level (e.g., correctly answering a few questions on a certification exam to verify awareness and sensitivity). We recognize that the process of becoming aware and respectful of diversity is not an endpoint that is achieved and then forgotten. In fact, treating cultural competence as a mere training objective can result in harm if competence is reduced to naïve stereotypes. Rather, cultural competence/cultural humility is a life-long developmental process.

Writing about cultural humility and physicians, Tervalon and Murray-García explain that

> It is a process that requires humility as individuals continually engage in self-reflection and self-critique as lifelong learners and reflective practitioners. It is a process that requires humility in how physicians bring into check the power imbalances that exist in the dynamics of physician-patient communication by using patient-focused interviewing and care. And it is a process that requires humility to develop and maintain mutually respectful and dynamic partnerships with communities on behalf of individual patients and communities in the context of community-based clinical and advocacy training models. (p. 118)

The concept of cultural humility applies equally well to midwifery care. Midwives have an ethical responsibility to become aware of their own cultural heritage and of the beliefs and practices of the communities they serve, and to cultivate the willingness to look beyond stereotypes to see clients as individuals.

There has also been a call to enrich the profession of midwifery through the recruitment and mentoring of diverse midwives (Kennedy, Erickson-Owens, & Davis, 2006). Ideally, the profession will be stronger and have greater capacity to serve diverse populations when fewer cultural discrepancies exist between midwives and clients. However, we do not mean to suggest here that an African American client is always best served by an African American midwife. Rather, all midwives should strive for self-reflective, developmental cultural humility that honors the diversity of each client. Consequently, cultural competence should be an objective of midwifery training and an area of continuing education for practicing midwives.

A HUMAN RIGHTS FRAMEWORK

Thompson (2004) has provided a unique perspective on ethics in midwifery by introducing a human rights perspective. By integrating concepts previously discussed in this book, such as informed choice and Kant's Ends Principle, with the treatment of women globally, Thompson makes a strong case for understanding midwifery care in the context of human rights. She promotes "a human rights framework for midwifery care that respects all persons, promotes informed decision making, takes measures to prevent any acts of violence or discrimination against clients, maintains privacy, and promotes safety for all midwifery care" (p. 175).

This model is based on adherence to "universal" principles, including justice and respect for dignity. Included under the umbrella of human rights are safe motherhood and reproductive rights. The pathway toward a human rights–

centered practice requires self-knowledge of one's values, ethics, and moral reasoning (Thompson, 2004). Thompson recommends knowledge of one's own values and culture, the practice of the golden rule, and understanding clients' values and culture to promote the human rights framework in midwifery care.

A human rights perspective acknowledges differences in culture and values, but also recognizes some common threads among those seeking maternity care. Carr and DeJoseph (2001) note that "all pregnant women have needs related to the fact that they are pregnant, but many women have further needs related to their economic, social, and ethnic circumstances and to their physical abilities, age, and sexual orientation" (p. 213). In this sense, culturally competent caregivers attend simultaneously to the universal and the unique. The mothers we serve are all seeking quality midwifery care, and we should treat them as pregnant women and mothers first, with honor and sensitivity of differences.

Thus far we have introduced the concepts of justice, diversity, and equity as multifaceted constructs. We recognized the importance of self-knowledge, cultural awareness, and acceptance and tolerance of those different from us. Next, we present case examples to further explore these ideas with realistic clinical scenarios. As you read the following cases, turn your attention to any stereotypes, biases, or preconceived notions you may have in response to the descriptions provided.

CASE EXAMPLES

CASE 1

Sandra and Julie, a lesbian couple, are expecting their first baby. At their initial prenatal visit, Rebecca, the midwife, is uncomfortable. After the appointment ends, Rebecca spends some time reflecting on the meeting. She believes that homosexuality is wrong and does not feel comfortable serving Sandra and Julie. However, she is aware that there are few midwives in the community, and that in all likelihood the couple would have a hard time finding a midwife in the area who is accepting of lesbian clients. Rebecca is inclined to call the couple and tell them that she is unable to serve them.

Questions

1. Does Rebecca have an ethical obligation to serve the couple?
2. How does Sandra and Julie's case relate to the concept of justice?
3. If Rebecca discontinues services with Sandra and Julie, what steps must be taken to ensure that the termination is conducted ethically?

Analysis

As mentioned earlier in this chapter, some midwifery organizations have incorporated notions of justice, equity, and respect for diversity in their ethical codes and statements. However, not all of these documents specifically address sexual orientation. Phrases such as "*all* members of society" and "the dignity of *all* people" suggest that respect is extended to individuals regardless of their sexual orientation, but this may not be universally accepted. In our diverse and pluralistic society, there are many who disapprove of homosexuality and bisexuality, often citing religious and moral reasons. Consistent with notions of cultural competence and cultural humility, Rebecca has taken an appropriate first step by reflecting on her own values and beliefs.

Rebecca might take time to reflect more deeply about her values as they relate to her professional activities as a midwife. For example, she might consider whether she is capable of providing quality care to a lesbian couple in spite of her disapproval of lesbianism. She might also explore the reasons behind her discomfort with nonheterosexual orientations and the extent to which stereotypes and cultural biases have shaped her own thoughts and feelings. If she has had limited experience with lesbian clients, she might pursue additional information to enhance her knowledge and understanding. Resources such as *The New Essential Guide to Lesbian Conception, Pregnancy, and Birth* (Brill, 2006) and *Health Care for Lesbians and Gay Men: Confronting Homophobia and Heterosexism* (Peterson, 1996) may be helpful in exploring relevant issues.

We must be clear in stating that Rebecca need not change her attitudes about homosexuality. Her beliefs and values are as important as those of her clients. However, she should consider broad ethical principles to guide her decision-making process. Justice, respect for the dignity of others, and nonmaleficence are all relevant to this example. Should she decide to terminate care, Rebecca must consider the impact of that decision on her clients. Simply referring them to another midwife who does not serve lesbians will not be in Sandra and Julie's best interest. If Rebecca decides to keep Sandra and Julie as clients but remains uncomfortable serving them, then she must assess the degree to which such discomfort interferes with her ability to provide quality care.

Perhaps the best course of action for Rebecca would be, following thorough self-reflection and consultation with colleagues, a frank and open discussion with Sandra and Julie about Rebecca's lack of experience serving lesbian clients, her values and beliefs, and hesitations about serving them. Such a conversation would provide Sandra and Julie with important information about their care (part of informed consent/choice) and open up the possibility of continuing care. One possible outcome is that Sandra and Julie disclose that they are accustomed to healthcare providers' discomfort and are willing to continue working with Rebecca so long as she is respectful and nondiscriminatory. Such openness may increase Rebecca's comfort and eliminate the need for her to discontinue services.

However, if Rebecca feels that she cannot provide adequate services to a lesbian couple, she should make every effort to make an appropriate referral to a qualified provider who is willing to work with lesbian couples (see Chapter 8 on referral). All women are entitled to high quality maternity care. As mentioned earlier, in this case there may not be an appropriate referral in Sandra and Julie's community. If that is true, Rebecca must consider other options and how they may affect the couple. Rebecca should continue to serve the couple until they establish care with another provider to prevent a gap in services. Additionally, Rebecca should terminate in such a way that is respectful to Sandra and Julie in an effort to minimize harm to them. If Rebecca works in a hospital or birth center, she should also consult the institution's nondiscrimination policies. Readers interested in this case may find Lasser and Gottlieb's (2004) discussion of ethical issues related to sexual orientation and psychotherapy helpful.

CASE 2

Anh is a Vietnamese woman who is two months pregnant. When asked by her midwife, Barbara, about her current health status, Anh reports that she has experienced painful headaches and has treated them with "coining," a traditional practice common in Southeast Asia that involves rubbing the skin with a coin and heated oil or a camphor-based ointment. Anh shows Barbara the red lines that were produced from the treatment on the back of her neck. When asked whether the treatment has been effective, Anh responds that it has been somewhat effective, but that the headaches persist. Barbara is unfamiliar with coining and is concerned about Anh's health and well-being.

Questions

1. How can Barbara apply her skills and training in Western midwifery care in a way that is compatible with Anh's traditional treatment?
2. What are the potential risks and benefits associated with deferring to Anh's judgment regarding treatment?
3. How do the concepts of cultural competence and cultural humility apply to this case?

Analysis

A good starting point for Barbara would be to educate herself about coining, and Anh may be an excellent source of information. With an open mind and an eagerness to learn, Barbara may ask Anh about the procedure, which ailments it is used to treat, and any other information that may be relevant (e.g., Anh's personal history with coining). Barbara may also consult experts in alternative medicine, as well as books and journal articles on the subject. The more information Barbara has, the better equipped she is to proceed with Anh's care.

Barbara may also try to assess the degree to which coining is an evidence-based treatment for headaches. One should not dismiss a treatment simply because it is a folk remedy, because many such cures are increasingly being subjected to scientific scrutiny (and some are demonstrating efficacy). That being said, risk and benefit must be taken very seriously. A treatment (alternative or medical) may have harmful side effects. An ineffective treatment that has no side effects may result in harm if the problem that it aims to treat persists. Additionally, medical treatments and alternative treatments jointly given may have unforeseen interactive effects. Only when Barbara gains more knowledge about the cultural practice of coining will she be able to address these concerns.

Barbara should be careful to respect Anh's beliefs and traditions. It would be inappropriate to dismiss coining as "an old wives' tale" or superstition. Barbara may instead see this as a learning opportunity and collaborate with Anh to understand her symptoms and chosen course of self-treatment. As a means of informed consent, Barbara should provide Anh with sufficient information about available treatment options that may be used in conjunction with or instead of coining so that Anh can make a good choice about her care (see Chapter 4 on informed choice/consent).

We must also be mindful of the fact that not all Vietnamese clients will practice coining, and that assumptions and stereotypes can result in harm as well. As Barbara explores traditional Southeast Asian healthcare practices, she will undoubtedly learn about other treatments in addition to coining. Although this information will inform her care of Anh and other Vietnamese clients, she must continue to treat each woman as an individual and respect not only her cultural heritage but also her unique life history, values, beliefs, and practices.

Case 3

Brenda and David have hired Liz, a homebirth midwife, but have had trouble meeting their financial obligations. Brenda is a stay-at-home mother of two, and David recently lost his job as a grocery store stocker. Liz has made adjustments to the couple's payment plan but has been concerned about their ability to pay the sliding-scale fee that was negotiated at the beginning of services. At a recent home visit, Liz became acutely aware of the couple's financial difficulties. She observed that there was very little food in the apartment, the electricity had been disconnected, and a stack of bills remained unopened. Liz is concerned about the family's well-being, their preparedness for the impending birth, and their ability to pay for their services. At times she feels that the family is a victim of economic misfortunes, but she also sometimes feels that the family has made poor financial decisions. She wants to discuss her concerns with Brenda and David but is unsure as to how she should begin. At their next appointment, Brenda and David shared with Liz their feelings of being judged for their economic situation.

Questions

1. How are poverty and socioeconomic status related to diversity, equity, and justice?
2. What is the significance of the midwife's concern about the underlying causes of the family's economic difficulties?
3. What are a midwife's obligations to a client who is unable to pay?

Analysis

Liz has genuine concern for Brenda and David and also wants to be sure that she is compensated for her services. Although she has achieved success and financial independence as a professional midwife, she had first hand experience of financial difficulties in her youth and relates to the challenges that Brenda and David are experiencing. After reflecting on her thoughts and feelings about her clients, Liz has come to realize that her attitude is shaped in part by the thought that "I worked hard and made good choices to achieve financial independence, but Brenda and David have not done the same." Liz is aware that this is an oversimplification, and that in reality, the circumstances and chains of events are far more complex.

After more careful consideration, Liz pays greater attention to factors independent of decision making and hard work, both in her life and Brenda's. Liz recalls the grandmother who paid off her student loans as a graduation gift; Brenda's aging father, who is in need of her daily care; and the added expense of purchases on credit for those who cannot afford to pay cash. Liz also reflects on Brenda and David's resilience in spite of their economic hardship; they have found creative ways to make ends meet to the best of their abilities.

Sociology has given a great deal of attention to a concept known as "the culture of poverty" (Lewis, 1968). Rather than characterizing the poor as deviant, incompetent, or ill-equipped, the culture of poverty addresses the subject "in a balanced way about the personal damage the poor sustain at the hands of a society that has ceased to care. Unlike other explanations of poverty, it concedes the poor have been damaged by the system but insists this damage does not clinically disqualify them from determining their own fate" (Harvey & Reed, 1996, p. 467). From this perspective, the poor have the internal resources to adapt to their circumstances.

As Liz continues to think about her clients, she begins to identify Brenda and David's strengths and assets. They are committed to having a healthy pregnancy and home birth, work hard to follow recommendations, attend their appointments on time, and come prepared with questions. Although her concerns about the family's well-being and ability to pay for services remain, Liz feels that her inventory of Brenda and David's internal assets has given her a fresh perspective.

Liz meets with Brenda and David at their next appointment. She opens by acknowledging all that appears to be going well, followed by her concerns in a frank and nonevaluative manner. Brenda and David share that although they initially felt judged, they have now been reminded that Liz is indeed supportive of them. Liz helps connect the family to social service agencies and a debt management service. They also resolve payment issues for their midwifery services by renegotiating a payment plan with Liz.

REFERENCES

American College of Nurse-Midwives (ACNM). (2008). *American College of Nurse-Midwives code of ethics with explanatory statements.* Silver Spring, MD: Author.

American Psychological Association (APA). (2002). *Ethical principles of psychologists and code of conduct.* Retrieved June 22, 2009, from http://www.apa.org/ethics/code2002.html

Beauchamp, T. L., & Childress, J. F. (2009). *Principles of biomedical ethics* (6th ed.). New York: Oxford University Press.

Boufford, J., & Lee, P. (2002). Health policy making: The role of the federal government. In M. Danis, C. Clancy, & L. Churchill (Eds.), *Ethical dimensions of health policy* (pp. 157–183). New York: Oxford University Press.

Brill, S. (2006). *The new essential guide to lesbian conception, pregnancy, and birth.* New York: Alyson Press.

Carr, C. A., & DeJoseph, J. F. (2001). Perinatal care among diverse populations of women. In L. V. Walsh (Ed.), *Midwifery: Community-based care during the childbearing years* (pp. 211–218). Philadelphia: W. B. Saunders.

Harrod, K. S., Hanson, L., & Osborne, K. (2007). Legislation and policy development. In L. A. Ament (Ed.), *Professional issues in midwifery* (pp. 147–173). Sudbury, MA: Jones and Bartlett.

Harvey, D. L., & Reed, M. H. (1996). The culture of poverty: An ideological analysis. *Sociological Perspectives, 39*(4), 465–495.

Hinman, L. M. (2008). *Ethics: A pluralistic approach to moral theory.* Belmont, CA: Thompson.

International Confederation of Midwives (ICM). (2003). *ICM international code of ethics for midwives.* Retrieved January 30, 2009, from http://www.internationalmidwives.org/Documentation/Coredocuments/tabid/322/Default.aspx

Jones, S. R. (2000). *Ethics in midwifery.* London: Mosby.

Kennedy, H. P., Erickson-Owens, D., & Davis, J. A. P. (2006). Voices of diversity in midwifery: A qualitative research study. *Journal of Midwifery and Women's Health, 51*(2), 85–90.

Lasser, J., & Gottlieb, M. (2004). Treating patients distressed regarding their sexual orientation: Clinical and ethical alternatives. *Professional Psychology: Research and Practice, 35*(2), 194–200.

Lewis, O. (1968). The culture of poverty. In D. P. Moynihan (Ed.), *On understanding poverty: Perspectives from the social sciences* (pp. 187–200). New York: Basic Books.

Midwives Alliance of North America (MANA). (1997). *Statement of values and ethics.* Washington, DC: Author.

Nursing and Midwifery Council. (2008). *The code: Standards of conduct, performance and ethics for nurses and midwives.* London: Author.

Paasche-Orlow, M. (2004). The ethics of cultural competence. *Academic Medicine, 79*(4), 347–350.

Peterson, K. J. (1996). *Health care for lesbians and gay men: Confronting homophobia and heterosexism.* New York: Routledge.

Rawls, J. (1971). *A theory of justice.* Cambridge, MA: Belknap Press of Harvard University Press.

Tervalon, M., & Murray-García, J. (1998). Cultural humility versus cultural competence: A critical distinction in defining physician training outcomes in multicultural education. *Journal of Health Care for the Poor and Underserved, 9*(2), 117–125.

Thompson, J. B. (2004). A human rights framework for midwifery care. *Journal of Midwifery and Women's Health, 49*(3), 175–181.

Williamson, M., & Harrison, L. (2001). Dealing with diversity: Incorporating cultural sensitivity into professional midwifery practice. *Australian Journal of Midwifery, 14*(4), 22–26.

Young, I. M. (1990). *Justice and the politics of difference.* Princeton, NJ: Princeton University Press.

CHAPTER 11

Addressing Ethical Concerns

UNETHICAL BEHAVIOR

If unethical behavior did not exist, there would be no need for ethical codes and standards (nor would there be a need for this book). Many questions about the ethical behavior of midwives remain unanswered. We do not know what kinds of ethical dilemmas are most common in midwifery. Nor do we know what midwives perceive as the most common ethical violations in the profession. The profession would benefit greatly from survey research that generated self-reported data on midwives and ethics. An anonymous survey might also shed light on the most frequently self-reported ethical violations. In the absence of such data, we must rely on anecdotal information that has been gathered unscientifically and therefore unsystematically. Nevertheless, the anecdotal evidence suggests that unethical behavior exists, although we do not know how pervasive or serious the violations may be. This chapter explores the idea of unethical behavior, provides some guidelines for responding to such behavior, and addresses ways that midwifery can promote better conduct.

Discussions of unethical behavior have the potential to raise strong emotional responses from professionals for a variety of reasons. Some may feel defensive of midwifery and express concerns that drawing attention to the unethical behavior of midwives tarnishes the public's perception of midwifery. This is understandable, given the documented efforts of physicians' organizations to discredit midwifery (see American College of Obstetricians and Gynecologists, 2008; American Medical Association, 2008). Others may be reluctant to talk about unethical behavior for fear that they will be scrutinized. Finally, confronting unethical behavior has the potential to cause rifts and conflict within the profession. Despite these concerns, addressing deviations from ethical standards is critical for consumer protection and the health and well-being of the profession.

In recent history there have been reports in the press about midwives who have practiced outside established ethical standards or the law, or both (e.g., "Illegal midwife," 1996). Additionally, many state midwifery boards establish and maintain public records of midwives cited for violations, and many of these can be found on the Internet. To fully understand the phenomenon of complaints and enforcement, one must address the context in which this process occurs. We believe that cultural beliefs related to personal responsibility coupled with highly litigious behavior represent significant contributing factors.

The idea of responsibility typically surfaces in political rhetoric. During the 2008 presidential campaign, candidates were frequently asked about the mortgage crisis. Responses invariably included discussions of predatory lenders and *personal responsibility*, as if to say that although banks were irresponsibly offering loans, consumers needed to exercise restraint. This theme emerges repeatedly in a government that tries to balance the need to protect citizens (e.g., the Food and Drug Administration's role in making sure that our food is safe) and the recognition that individuals have the capacity to exercise judgment and care for themselves (e.g., to be thoughtful about our eating choices).

There are two sides to the coin of responsibility. On the one hand, the concept is used to limit social welfare programs with arguments that individuals should "pull themselves up by their bootstraps." Individuals are also expected to take responsibility for their actions. On the other hand, advocates of tort reform argue that frivolous lawsuits are a product of individuals failing to take responsibility for their actions and displacing blame onto care providers. For example, an individual who opts for elective surgery to correct his vision and is informed of the risks may sue the surgeon who performed the procedure correctly. Rather than accepting responsibility for taking a risk, the patient asks the physician to accept responsibility.

We acknowledge the complexity of these issues and recognize that in many cases, responsibility for health is shared by patients and providers, rendering the "his fault/her fault" distinction moot. We also understand that some complaints against providers are legitimate and serve an important role in maintaining consumer protections and the provision of quality care. The marginalization of midwives, discussed in Chapter 1, also factors into our discussion. Already on the defensive as medical associations work to limit the practice of midwifery, midwives may feel particularly vulnerable. This perspective likely shapes midwives' beliefs and attitudes about complaints and enforcement processes.

Unethical behavior must be taken very seriously, primarily in the interest of preventing harm and maximizing benefit to clients. We also emphasize the importance of developing and maintaining trust in the profession, because the public's perception of and confidence in midwifery is critical. Ultimately, we seek to transcend mere compliance with laws and codes such that we provide high-quality, ethical care to women and their families (Thompson, 2003).

REASONS FOR UNETHICAL BEHAVIOR

There are many reasons why midwives may behave unethically. Sometimes ethics violations are simply a factor of misunderstanding ethical standards or of a lack of awareness. For example, a midwife may wrongfully assume that the standards concerning multiple relationships are limited to those in which the nonmidwifery relationship is financial in nature. Such misunderstandings are relatively easy to address informally, and most midwives who are aware of and understand the guidelines will follow them. Sometimes midwives find themselves facing an ethical dilemma and feel that they are in a Catch-22; regardless of the path selected for resolution, some ethical standard will be violated. Others may behave unethically because they are experiencing psychological problems that impair their decision-making skills. No matter what the reason for the unethical behavior, such problems must be addressed.

ADDRESSING THE UNETHICAL BEHAVIOR OF OTHERS

Over the course of a midwife's career, she will likely encounter the ethical misconduct of other midwives. We recognize that addressing the unethical behavior of our colleagues may be challenging, but it is vital for consumer protection and the maintenance of professional standards in midwifery. We offer the following example to further explore the issue of approaching another midwife about ethical concerns.

Brenda asks her midwife, Charise, to falsely report the date of birth on the certificate so that her baby will not have to share her husband's birthday. Charise explains that falsification of records is illegal and unethical and refuses to comply. Brenda insists that it must be legitimate, because her last midwife, Angel, changed the birth date of Brenda's first child. Charise now knows that her colleague has engaged in unethical and illegal behavior. What should Charise do about this?

Charise could file a complaint against Angel to the state midwifery board and the state agency that maintains vital records. However, this would be premature and inappropriate, given the little information that was provided to Charise. Perhaps Brenda lied about Angel's behavior in an effort to pressure Charise to comply with the request. If Angel did not act inappropriately, a complaint filed against her could cause her great distress and require her to expend time, money, and energy defending herself. False allegations also waste the time of governing boards.

Another option for Charise is to ignore Brenda's report. Charise may not take Brenda seriously, or may choose to ignore the allegation in the interest of protecting her colleague and friend. If the allegations are true and Charise chooses to ignore the problem, Angel may continue to engage in illegal and unethical behavior (which could result in harm). Alternatively, Charise may believe that Angel engages in misconduct but chooses not to address the concern because she believes it is none of her business. As a result, she may think less of Angel and cease to send her referrals without even knowing whether she engaged in inappropriate behavior.

A third option, and the best choice, is for Charise to approach Angel directly. There are many benefits to this course of action. By approaching Angel with the concern, Charise demonstrates respect for Angel as a colleague and a person. If Angel had falsified records, she might be unaware that her actions were inappropriate. Angel might then take corrective action and discontinue the practice of falsifying birth dates when requested by clients. Or by discussing the concern with Angel, Charise may learn that the client's report was false. All of these outcomes are superior to filing a complaint or ignoring the client's report.

In some instances, a midwife may continue to act unethically even after the problem has been brought to her attention. Should the problem persist following informal efforts to address the concern, a formal process should follow (e.g., filing a complaint with a licensing board or ethics committee). The formal process is a legitimate vehicle for addressing the problem, but should be considered only after the informal steps have been tried. The informal process also can be conceptualized as a screening tool and information-gathering step in addressing concerns. In many cases, this step will resolve the issue without unnecessary involvement of third parties.

Following a formal complaint and investigation, an ethics committee or board may dismiss the charges as proven to be unfounded or may enforce a wide range of sanctions and directives, including fines, mandatory supervision and continuing education in ethics, censure, corrective actions, suspension or loss of license, and expulsion from a professional organization. Individuals about whom a complaint has been filed may also receive an educative letter that is designed to prevent the problem from occurring again (Koocher & Keith-Spiegel, 1998).

There may be cases in which the unethical behavior presents imminent danger to clients and should not follow the sequence just described (i.e., informally approaching the person who is suspected of unethical behavior and then later filing a formal complaint). In such cases, swift action should be taken to prevent serious harm while maintaining respect for the dignity of those involved. Case 3 at the end of this chapter addresses this situation.

Another critical step in addressing the unethical behavior of others is documenting the process in writing. Documentation creates a record of your responsible actions should you be asked how you addressed the concern (e.g., in legal proceedings). Documentation should be handled securely, like any other confidential record. The recording of the process may be as simple as the following examples:

August 31, 2009
Met with Louise Brown, CPM, at her office and shared with her that my new client, TJ, reported that Louise had terminated care abruptly without provisions for trans-

fer of care. Louise acknowledged a lapse in judgment, offered to take responsibility for her actions, and stated that she would issue an apology to TJ. She made a commitment to exercise better judgment in the termination of care in the future.

September 19, 2009
At the community swimming pool today I heard Debbie Patterson, CNM, talking about her clients with other swimmers. She was disclosing confidential information. I spoke with her privately about the importance of maintaining confidentiality. She dismissed my concerns and insisted that there's no harm in talking about clients' births. I informed her that breaking confidentiality is a serious ethical violation and she stated that she will continue to tell birth stories with identifying information, indicating that the stories "need to be heard." After leaving the pool I contacted the state midwifery board and filed a formal complaint. I was issued reference #45621 for the complaint.

Note that in both of these examples, the midwife documents the unethical behavior, as well as the steps that were taken to address the unethical behavior. We are not suggesting that midwives police one another with a punitive attitude. Rather, we see the informal and formal processes of addressing ethical concerns as an example of professionalism and self-regulation in the place of external regulation (see Chapter 1). Also, note that the formal complaint comes only after informal steps have been tried.

Filing a formal complaint typically leads to an investigation and, should the investigation conclude that a practitioner violated ethical standards, some form of enforcement (e.g., fines, mandatory continuing education in ethics, suspension or revocation of license). Licensing boards are not universally effective at enforcing such rules. For example, in 2009 the California Board of Registered Nursing became headline news following reports that allegedly dangerous nurses continued to practice even after complaints were filed (Medical News Today, 2009). If the role of a state board is to protect the public by regulating practice, professionals must ensure that the board is effective in carrying out its mission.

Presently, most of the major midwifery professional organizations do not directly address the ways in which midwives should respond to alleged ethical misconduct. Although not a code of ethics, the Candidate Information Bulletin of the North American Registry of Midwives (NARM) includes a grievance mechanism (Figure 11-1). The process described by NARM serves a purpose more general than addressing ethical concerns and was designed for complaints against midwives. NARM provides Certified Professional Midwives (or applicants) with "the opportunity to speak to any written complaints against them before any action is taken against their certificate (or application)" (NARM, 2008, p. 57). However, NARM's mechanism begins with efforts to resolve concerns with a local peer review rather than a formal complaint. NARM provides detailed recommendations to guide the peer review process. Should the peer review fail to successfully resolve the problem, a formal complaint to the NARM board is filed.

Figure 11-1   NARM's grievance mechanism: flow of activity.

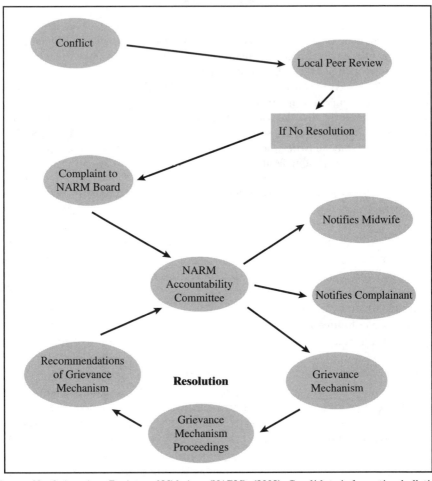

Source: North American Registry of Midwives (NARM). (2008). *Candidate information bulletin.*
Retrieved July 15, 2009, from http://www.narm.org/certification.htm

Formal, written procedures for addressing ethical concerns provide midwives and clients with a fair and just way of dealing with problems when they arise. Ultimately, these procedures must balance respect for midwives' autonomy and dignity with consumer protection to ensure that there are fair and just ways of approaching questionable or unethical conduct. It is our hope that future revisions of the major ethical codes will provide more guidance to midwives to ensure that concerns about ethical conduct are taken seriously, offering systematic guidelines to address unethical behavior, and reflecting standards of justice and dignity.

ADDRESSING ONE'S OWN UNETHICAL BEHAVIOR

Earlier we acknowledged that approaching another midwife about questionable conduct might be challenging. Addressing one's own unethical behavior may be just as difficult, if not more so. When we realize that we have violated ethical standards, we might feel embarrassed, ashamed, or less than competent. Some may entertain the fantasy that the error in judgment will disappear if ignored. Others may engage in further unethical behavior, such as lying, to hide misdeeds. Ultimately, the best course of action is to take responsibility.

Taking responsibility for one's mistakes involves several steps. First, one must acknowledge to oneself that one has acted unethically. Second, one must take concrete steps to take corrective action. This may include apologies, reparations, and implementation of an improvement plan. We use the following example to illustrate this process of taking responsibility.

Lara is a nurse–midwife employed by a large urban hospital. In an effort to save time when work gets busy and hectic, Lara has cut some corners with the informed consent process by asking patients to sign consent documents without fully explaining them. On a particularly stressful shift, a patient complained that she did not feel like she was actively participating in making informed choices about her care. The complaint brought the lapse to Lara's attention.

In an effort to take full responsibility, Lara apologized to the patient and validated her concern. She acknowledged that the informed consent process was rushed and consequently was "mere consent" rather than truly *informed* consent. Lara told the patient that she accepted full responsibility and gave the patient an opportunity to revisit the consent process, this time more thoroughly. Lara made a commitment to attend a continuing education workshop on ethics and make time for informed consent with patients in the future. She also documented this process for her own records. Were someone to file a complaint against Lara, she would be able to demonstrate a good-faith effort to take responsibility and corrective action. She may also use this as an opportunity to review the hospital's policies with her colleagues and supervisors in an effort to improve the informed consent process for all.

Thus far we have focused our attention in this chapter on the ways in which we respond or react when we become aware of unethical behavior. We shift our focus now to ways in which midwifery can promote ethical behavior and actively prevent ethical problems from occurring.

PROACTIVE ETHICS

Ethical standards in most professions develop reactively, which is to say that codes are written to address existing concerns. For example, as the use of computers became more widespread, many professional organizations added elements to their codes of ethics that addressed ethical concerns regarding electronic communication, confidentiality of electronic records, and so forth. The reactive approach responds to ethical problems as they emerge, but does little to prevent new problems from surfacing.

We endorse a proactive approach to professional ethics that aims to anticipate ethical concerns of the future and work toward preventing them. This may seem paradoxical, for we have no crystal ball to foresee the ethical challenges of tomorrow. Nevertheless, we have sufficient information about current trends to anticipate shifts in maternity care in the coming years. Consider the following: major efforts to overhaul health care in the United States, increasing legal support for gay/lesbian marriage, advances in fertility and reproductive technologies, and demographic shifts in the ethnic/cultural composition of the country. All of these signs of change present an opportunity to think proactively about our ethical standards so that we can plan and create ethical standards that serve us for the future.

Another critical element of a reflective approach to ethics in midwifery involves inquiry and research. The work of Faye Thompson (2004) serves as an extraordinary example of focusing a scientific eye on ethics in midwifery. Unless we ask questions about and seek answers regarding ethics and midwives, we will practice with insufficient information, experience obstacles to successful resolution, and have little knowledge of factors that facilitate positive outcomes. Do midwives follow a structured sequence of decision-making steps when faced when ethical dilemmas? If not, then how do they make their decisions? Which steps lead to successful resolutions? We strongly advocate for more research in this fundamental domain of practice.

PRESERVICE TRAINING AND CONTINUING EDUCATION

Central to the education of aspiring midwives is the acquisition of the knowledge and skills that are the backbone of midwifery training and practice. A more subtle, yet equally important, component of midwifery training is the socialization process that transmits cultural knowledge to future midwives. Through the course of her training, while the student of midwifery learns practical skills she also becomes acculturated to the Midwives Model of Care (MMOC) (Rothman, 1979) and the culture of midwifery. She also begins to develop an understanding of (and internalization of) what Thompson (2004) calls an ethic of midwifery.

There are many paths to becoming a midwife (Tritten & Southern, 2002), and these routes vary in their emphasis on ethics. Some courses of study contain a standalone class in ethics for midwives, whereas others have little to no training in the area of ethics. We strongly advocate for preservice training in ethics for all midwifery students. Midwives need a clear understanding of ethical codes and standards, common ethical challenges, and processes for addressing ethical concerns when they arise. Without such preparation, students of midwifery will be ill-equipped to face the challenges that will undoubtedly present themselves over the course of their careers.

Midwives in training should have opportunities to read and study the ethical codes and then apply what they have learned to realistic case scenarios. They should be able to read case examples and identify the ethical standards or issues that are at the core of the situations (e.g., to recognize that informed choice is the underlying concern when a midwife fails to disclose potential risks of a procedure to a client). Students of midwifery should also learn problem-solving approaches and be able to apply them to sample ethical dilemmas to demonstrate their ability to think through difficult decisions (see Chapter 12). Clearly, these learning objectives cannot be covered in a brief lecture or as a short unit in a professional issues class. Rather, ethics deserves a significant amount of time and attention proportional to its importance.

Ethics education should not be limited to professionals in training. In fact, other human service professions require continuing education in ethics (e.g., licensed psychologists in Texas must have at least three hours of ethics training every year). There are many reasons for providing ethics education for the licensed/certified professional. As discussed in Chapter 1, ethics are continually evolving as the landscape of practice changes. Technology, law, and professional standards do not remain static. Consequently, the training in ethics that one received as a student of midwifery is likely to lose relevance over time. The professional midwife who is committed to the highest standards of ethical care will regard ethics training as a life-long pursuit.

As we demonstrate in Chapter 12, ethics in midwifery is more than a book or a course. The professional midwife actively engages in ethical thinking on a daily basis and needs opportunities to reflect on "doing ethics" and to stay abreast of current trends, innovations, and updates with respect to applied ethics in midwifery. Additionally, continuing education in ethics provides midwives with the newest revisions of ethical codes and standards. Members of professional organizations such the American College of Nurse-Midwives (ACNM), the Midwives Alliance of North America (MANA), and the International Confederation of Midwives (ICM) may also have opportunities to provide input that will shape the codes of the future.

CODE REVISION AS PROACTIVE ETHICS

Typically, ethical codes and standards are written for the present. Taking into consideration the current professional issues and needs, the authors of codes work hard to craft documents that are useful to the profession. Over time, revisions become necessary to address changes in the field. Unfortunately, much of this revision process is reactive rather than proactive, which is to say that the codes are revised in response to the new developments. Ideally, code revision should serve a proactive function such that it anticipates tomorrow's ethical challenges and provides professionals with parameters of behavior regarding such changes. Naturally, prediction of what is to come can be difficult, but it is certainly worth the effort because it enhances the profession's capacity to adapt to new ethical concerns. We are mindful that, although the codes are critical, they are only a starting point. Ultimately, we aim "to inspire ethical practice from within the individual rather than mere compliance with professional codes and employer policies" (Thompson, 2003, p. 599).

Proactive ethics involves staying abreast of new developments in the field, as well as historical events that may impact care. Ethical education is most effective when it builds upon a foundation that was laid during training, and we advocate for ethical training for all student midwives. Continuing education in ethics is essential for midwives to maintain ethical practice, and more to the point, to practice ethical thinking. As midwives develop consensus around ethical practice, ethical codes reflect these advances.

To conclude this chapter, we offer case examples that illustrate how midwives faced with complex concerns about unethical behavior use a process of addressing their concerns in a positive manner that aims to respect the dignity of all parties involved. Following each case example, we provide questions to consider and some analysis of the example.

CASE EXAMPLES

CASE 1

Meryl had been practicing as a Certified Professional Midwife (CPM) for three years before she took on Sasha as her apprentice. The two found their working relationship to be productive and harmonious and agreed to become business partners once Sasha became fully licensed. They formed a partnership and named their new enterprise "Harmony Midwifery." Unfortunately, after six months of collaborating as colleagues, their relationship begins to sour.

Sasha has confided in friends her feeling that Meryl continues to treat her like an apprentice rather than as an equal. She also suspects that Meryl has discouraged new clients from working with Sasha, because she heard from a third party that Meryl has described her as "less experienced and less qualified." Sasha feels hurt and offended that Meryl has apparently treated her poorly and without the dignity and respect that should be offered to a colleague.

Unbeknownst to Sasha, Meryl has harbored some unspoken concerns about Sasha's competence and readiness for clients who may present unusual or highly challenging clinical issues. Meryl has had the opportunity to participate in Sasha's training and has observed her knowledge and skills develop over time. Meryl also believes that her training in another state was superior to Sasha's training and that she is justified in steering some clients away from Sasha until she gains more experience. Although she agreed to start a new business with Sasha as a partner, Meryl still thinks that Sasha has a lot to learn. Meryl has shared her concerns with other experienced midwives.

Questions

1. What key ethical principles or standards are at the heart of Meryl and Sasha's problem?
2. What are the advantages and disadvantages of an informal approach to resolution?
3. If you were asked to serve as a third-party mediator for Meryl and Sasha, how would you facilitate a productive discussion?

Analysis

Working effectively as a partner with another midwife can present challenges linked to a variety of ethical standards. Meryl and Sasha began their relationship in the context of an apprenticeship that was inherently unequal; Meryl was in a supervisory role. However, the relationship eventually became one of peers as they entered into a new business venture as two professional midwives. The fact that Meryl and Sasha have not clearly communicated their thoughts and feelings about their new working relationship exacerbates the underlying concerns.

Both Sasha and Meryl should have made an effort to communicate with each other before going to other midwives about their perceptions of the problem.

Although it is certainly advisable to consult with colleagues about ethical concerns, great care must be taken to avoid gossip or disclosures that could result in harm. Consequently, all peer ethics consultations should be confidential and anonymous if possible. In short, Meryl and Sasha need to express their thoughts and feelings to one another.

Optimally, a conversation about the problem will result in a resolution that satisfies both parties. For example, they may come to an understanding that each has a different level of training and unique skill set and makes significant contributions to the practice. An outcome of the conversation may be the development of an equitable way of assigning new clients to each midwife. They may also agree to discontinue negative talk about each other to clients and other midwives.

In this case example, Meryl and Sasha attempt to resolve their problem informally. Of course, efforts to resolve such conflicts informally may fail. The use of a neutral, third-party mediator may be helpful in guiding Meryl and Sasha toward resolution. Peer review may also be in order. Midwives working for large institutions such as hospitals may have systems in place, perhaps through an ombudsman, to facilitate conflict resolution. Should these efforts fail, midwives may file formal complaints or grievances to address the problem.

If either Meryl or Sasha decides to file a formal complaint or grievance, she should be able to put her concerns in writing such that they are clear, objective, and linked to practice and/or ethical standards. For example, in a complaint filed with the American College of Nurse-Midwives, Sasha can cite the ACNM's (2008) ethical code, which states:

> In negotiating the tension between "self" and "other," midwives have to balance their need for professional autonomy and recognition of their knowledge and skills with the competing needs for autonomy of the "other," be that a client, administrator or colleague who maintains a different perspective. Such cases require a delicate balancing act, often aided by some reframing of both positions. (p. 4)

Once a complaint is filed, the organization that receives the complaint will investigate and enforce penalties as warranted. Again, we endorse informal conflict resolution as the first step and encourage professionals to pursue formal complaint as a last resort.

CASE 2

Iris Jenkins, a certified nurse–midwife (CNM) at Presbyterian Hospital, works closely with Tim Kurz, an obstetrician. Over the past several months, Tim has been making unwanted comments of a sexual nature to Iris. More recently, Tim's behavior has escalated to include inappropriate emails to Iris and, on one occasion, an inappropriate touch. Iris initially found Tim's behavior annoying, but the emails and touch have made her very uncomfortable. Iris feels that her work environment is intimidating and that Tim's behavior is interfering with her work.

Iris has asked other midwives and nurses about Tim's behavior and has received a range of feedback. Some have encouraged her to keep quiet in the interest of preserving her job. Others have shared similar experiences but reported feeling helpless about the situation. Still others have reported that he treats them kindly and with respect. Uncertain about how to proceed, Iris takes her concerns to a counselor through the hospital's Employee Assistance Program (EAP).

The EAP counselor informs Iris, based on the description provided, that Tim's behavior sounds like sexual harassment. She advises Iris to approach Tim directly to tell him that his behavior is unwanted, inappropriate, and needs to end. Iris communicates her fear of losing her job and her feelings of intimidation, but the counselor helps her to develop the courage to confront Tim through role play scenarios.

The following week, Iris schedules an appointment with Tim. At the meeting, she tells him that he has behaved poorly and insists that he discontinue the inappropriate comments, emails, and touching. Tim responds with a dismissive laugh, tells Iris that she has an "active imagination," and walks out of the meeting. Deflated, Iris regrets talking to him about the problem and grows despondent. She schedules a follow-up appointment with her EAP counselor, but does not feel that it will do much good.

Meanwhile, Iris places a phone call to her state midwifery association for further guidance. She is informed that the state (and national) midwifery organizations only have the authority to enforce rules on their own members. Because Tim is not a member of the state midwifery organization, he cannot be subject to the associations' enforcement. Feeling that her options have been exhausted, Iris resigns and begins looking for another job.

Questions

1. Which ethical standards or codes did Tim violate in his interactions with Iris?
2. Other than her colleagues, EAP counselor, and state midwifery association, what other resources are available to Iris?
3. If midwifery organizations cannot accept complaints against Tim, who can?

Analysis

Although Iris did not use the term in her consultations with others, she was experiencing *sexual harassment*. According to the U.S. Equal Employment Opportunity Commission (EEOC),

> Unwelcome sexual advances, requests for sexual favors, and other verbal or physical conduct of a sexual nature constitute sexual harassment when this conduct explicitly or implicitly affects an individual's employment, unreasonably interferes with an individual's work performance, or creates an intimidating, hostile, or offensive work environment. (EEOC, 2009, para. 2)

The EAP counselor's advice was consistent with that provided by the EEOC: approach Tim directly and tell him to stop. However, Tim's failure to take responsibility for his behavior does not in any way suggest that Iris has no further options. Iris can file a formal grievance through the hospital, and she can also report Tim's behavior to any physicians' organization to which he belongs (e.g., the American Medical Association, the state medical board). The hospital, medical board, and physicians' organizations have the authority to address Tim's behavior. Iris can also file a complaint with the EEOC (for filing information, see http://www.eeoc.gov/facts/howtofil.html).

This case example highlights a problem that is both unethical and illegal: sexual harassment. As we have mentioned before, detailed discussion of legal issues in midwifery is beyond the scope of this text. However, we wish to draw attention to the fact that in some cases, unethical behavior may have legal ramifications. Midwives should be aware of the various mechanisms available for addressing unethical behavior.

CASE 3

Two university researchers, in collaboration with Springdale Hospital, have started a research project to analyze data from obstetric emergencies in three counties in hopes of identifying trends and patterns. Alice Clements, a CNM employed by Springfield Hospital, works with the university researchers by pulling the records of the emergency cases and removing identifying information. The university researchers do not have access to the confidential data. The research has been approved by the institutional review boards of both the university and the hospital, which is to say that the research has met established ethical standards.

As Alice goes through the process of removing identifying information from the charts, she notices that several emergency admissions came from a local, freestanding birthing center. She also found several cases from this center in which induction drugs were used. She was surprised that the midwives did not accompany the clients to the hospital during transport. Alarmed by this pattern, Alice immediately contacts the state midwifery board to report the unethical behavior of the midwives at the birthing center.

Questions

1. Does Alice have sufficient information to conclude that midwives at the birthing center behaved unethically?
2. If the birthing center midwives behaved unethically, what ethical standards were violated?
3. How might Alice's role as research collaborator affect her ethical decision making?

Analysis

Up until this point in the chapter, we have advocated for initially addressing unethical behavior through an informal approach. Were we to recommend this to Alice, we would advise her to contact the director of the birthing center. However, this case stands apart from the others in that it involves dangerous practices that must be addressed immediately. The slow process of informal mediation could waste precious time, putting other women at serious risk.

Administration of induction drugs outside a hospital setting puts women and fetuses at great risk. A freestanding birthing center that routinely induces its clients with drugs violates the foundations of bioethics: beneficence and nonmaleficence. Dangerous practices must circumvent the traditional approach of informal resolution in the interest of protecting clients and eliminating the use of unnecessarily risky interventions.

We should not underestimate the potential negative consequences of reporting directly to the state midwifery board. If Alice has misperceived the data and the birthing center midwives have in fact behaved ethically, the investigation may result in psychological distress, gossip, and distrust. As with any ethical dilemma, Alice must weigh the potential risks and benefits of any action and the impact on all parties involved (Thompson, 2007).

Reporting the birth center to the midwifery board could result in a rapid resolution to the problem, but this may not necessarily be the case. Recall that the California nursing board reportedly failed to respond to complaints against nurses in a timely manner (Medical News Today, 2009). Nevertheless, Alice must take immediate action to the best of her abilities. Even if the boards responsible for enforcement do not act swiftly, Alice still has an ethical obligation to report dangerous practices. She may also communicate directly with the birthing center by informing them that she has filed a complaint.

REFERENCES

American College of Nurse-Midwives (ACNM). (2008). *American College of Nurse-Midwives code of ethics with explanatory statements*. Silver Spring, MD: Author.

American College of Obstetricians and Gynecologists. (2008). *ACOG statement on home births*. Retrieved July 5, 2008, from http://www.acog.org/from_home/publications/press_releases /nr02-06-08-2.cfm

American Medical Association (AMA). (2008). *House of Delegates resolution 204*. Retrieved July 5, 2008, from http://www.ama-assn.org/ama/pub/category/18587.html

Equal Employment Opportunity Commission. (2009). *Sexual harassment*. Retrieved August 9, 2009, from http://www.eeoc.gov/laws/types/sexual_harassment.cfm

Illegal midwife. (1996, June 13). *The Victoria Advocate*, p. A2.

Koocher, G. P., & Keith-Spiegel, P. (1998). *Ethics in psychology: Professional standards and cases*. New York: Oxford University Press.

Medical News Today. (2009, July 15). *Schwarzenegger fires three California nursing board members*. Retrieved July 15, 2009, from http://www.medicalnewstoday.com/articles/157563.php

North American Registry of Midwives (NARM). (2008). *Candidate information bulletin*. Retrieved July 15, 2009, from http://www.narm.org/certification.htm

Rothman, B. K. (1979). *Two models in maternity care: Defining and negotiating reality*. New York: New York University Press.

Thompson, F. E. (2003). The practice setting: Site of ethical conflict for some mothers and midwives. *Nursing Ethics, 10*(6), 588–601.

Thompson, F. E. (2004). *Mothers and midwives: The ethical journey*. London: Books for Midwives.

Thompson, J. E. (2007). Professional ethics. In L. A. Ament (Ed.), *Professional issues in midwifery* (pp. 277–300). Sudbury, MA: Jones and Bartlett.

Tritten, J., & Southern, J. (2002). *Paths to becoming a midwife: Getting an education*. Eugene, OR: Midwifery Today.

CHAPTER 12

Ethical Thinking, Caring, and Decision Making

ETHICAL DECISION MAKING

A number of ethical decision-making models have relevance for healthcare professionals, the majority of which involve identifying a concern, applying ethical principles, examining alternatives, deciding on appropriate actions, and evaluating results. These tools are valuable for critically thinking about ethical dilemmas. They are compatible with and supplementary to the applied ethics that we have used in this book thus far. Ethical decision-making models have a specific application for healthcare providers. They guide the practitioner in a systematic approach to ethical problem solving. They are helpful in identifying ethical problems and providing directions to address ethical concerns, but on their own they do not adequately capture the social complexity of ethical dilemmas, with their relational and contextual considerations (Tschudin, 2003).

Ethical decision-making models lack the social aspects of human cognition and behavior. Like principle-based ethics, these models are oversimplistic and are limited in expressing the contextual nature of ethical dilemmas. Yet this does not reduce their usefulness to clinicians, especially if the practitioner understands the gestalt, or big picture, within which ethical behavior occurs. Models are like other tools: to use them correctly, one must understand their limits. The myth of impartiality is another major shortcoming of the current models (Lützén, 1997). No practitioner can maintain objectivity at the level that is suggested by the authors of these tools. We are embedded in our work environments, relationships, and cultural contexts to too great an extent to have impartiality. For instance, a midwife working for a military hospital is also employed by the U.S. Armed Forces. She is enmeshed in military organization, culture, and protocols. These will inform her practice and influence her ethics. A skilled clinician should attempt to maintain awareness of biases and verbalize them to clients when appropriate, but she cannot rid herself of these biases, nor can she think or act with complete objectivity, although that may be the goal.

We briefly examine two bioethical decision-making models for their usefulness and limitations. We have chosen them based on their applicability to midwifery. Many midwives are familiar with the model developed by Thompson and Thompson and updated in 2004, because it is widely referenced in midwifery literature (Thompson, 2007). The second model is highly recommended for use in nursing (Thompson, Melia, & Boyd, 2005).

The Thompson and Thompson Bioethical Decision-Making Model outlines a step-by-step process by which midwives and other healthcare professionals solve and evaluate ethical dilemmas (Table 12-1). The first three steps involve gathering data and identifying ethical concerns. Diverse viewpoints and cultural meanings are considered. The next three steps involve values and moral positions, with an emphasis on self-awareness and tolerance of diverse perspectives. Steps 7 through 9 are concerned with making a decision—with careful consideration of each party's role, the range of potential solutions, and the possible outcomes of each—and planning a course of action. The final step is evaluation. Each step entails guidelines that require an impressive amount of time, clarity, and thoughtfulness. "It requires critical thinking, reflection, time, caring, integrity, and use of moral reasoning to sort out the key aspects of the situation, alternatives for action, and moral mandates from professional codes that can provide direction to the decision-making" (Thompson, 2007, p. 291). Thompson and Thompson's model is highly individualized, written as if the care provider could step outside of the contexts in which she or he works to review, identify, determine, and decide. The model is valuable as a problem-solving tool, but it does not capture the relational nature of ethical decisions in midwifery practice.

The DECIDE Model for Ethical Decision Making similarly engages the practitioner in identifying causal factors and includes contextual considerations alongside ethical principles (Thompson, Melia, & Boyd, 2005). First, the practi-

---

Table 12-1   Thompson & Thompson's Bioethical Decision-Making Model

Step 1:	**Review the situation** to determine: 1. Health problems – physical, spiritual, mental, psychosocial. 2. Decision/actions needed immediately & in near future. 3. Ethical components of situation and decision/action. 4. Key individuals potentially affected by the decision/action & outcomes. 5. Any potential human rights violations in situation.
Step 2:	**Gather additional information** to clarify and understand: 1. Legal constraints, if any. 2. Limited time to thoroughly explore. 3. Decision capacity of individual(s). 4. Institutional policies that affect choices in situation. 5. Values inherent in choice of information.

Table 12-1   Thompson & Thompson's Bioethical Decision-Making Model
(continued)

Step 3:	**Identify the ethical issues or concerns** in the situation: 1. Name the ethical concern. 2. Explore historical roots of each. 3. Identify current philosophical/religious positions on each issue. 4. Discuss societal/cultural views on each issue.
Step 4:	**Define personal and professional moral positions** on ethical concerns: 1. Review personal biases/constraints on issues raised. 2. Understand personal values affected by situation/ethical issues raised. 3. Review professional codes of ethics (moral behavior) for guidance. 4. Identify any conflicting loyalties and/or obligations of professionals and family in the situation. 5. Think about your level of moral development operant in this situation. 6. Identify the virtues needed for professional action.
Step 5:	**Identify moral positions of key individuals** in the situation: 1. Think about levels of moral development operant in each participant. 2. Identify any communication gaps or misunderstandings. 3. Provide guidance in clarifying varying levels of moral development.
Step 6:	**Identify value conflicts,** if any: 1. Provide guidance in identifying potential conflicts, interests, competing values. 2. Work toward possible resolution of conflict based on respect for differences. 3. Seek consultation if needed to resolve key conflicts.
Step 7:	**Determine who should make needed decision:** 1. Clarify your role in the situation. 2. Who 'owns' the problem/decision? 3. Who stands to lose or gain the most from the decision/action? 4. Is the decision to be made by single individual or group?
Step 8:	**Identify the range of actions with anticipated outcomes of each:** 1. Determine the moral justification for each potential action. 2. Identify the ethical theory that supports each action. 3. Apply concepts of beneficence and fairness to each potential action. 4. Attach outcomes to each potential action and determine best outcome. 5. Are additional actions/decisions required as a result of each action?

(continues)

Table 12-1   Thompson & Thompson's Bioethical Decision-Making Model
(continued)

Step 9:	**Decide on a course of action and carry it out:** 1. Understand why a given action was chosen. 2. Help all involved understand these reasons. 3. Establish a time frame for review of the decision/action and expected outcomes. 4. Determine who can best carry out the chosen action/decision.
Step 10:	**Evaluate/review outcomes of decisions/actions:** 1. Determine whether expected outcomes occurred. 2. Is a new decision or action needed? 3. Was the decision process fair and complete? 4. What was the response to the action by each key individual? 5. What did you learn from this situation?

Source: "Professional Ethics," by J. E. Thompson, in L. A. Ament (Ed.), 2007, *Professional Issues in Midwifery* (Sudbury, MA: Jones and Bartlett), pp. 290–291. Reprinted with permission.

tioner defines the problem and identifies relevant ethical principles. Then, she or he considers the possible options and expected outcomes of each. Finally, the practitioner decides on an appropriate action, acts, and evaluates the outcome. The model goes into little detail about the nature of these contextual factors, but offers recognition of their influence on the ethical dilemma. Overall, it is a simpler approach to ethical problem solving than Thompson and Thompson's (Thompson, 2007) model. Whether that is an asset or liability may depend on the nature of the dilemma at hand. Some situations may require a more gradual, systematic approach than others.

The aforementioned models are built on ethical principles. Principle-based ethical theory is the backbone of both ethical decision-making models and codes of ethics (see Chapter 2). There are numerous criticisms of this approach, including oversimplicity, prescriptiveness, and reductionism. *Reductionism* implies a philosophical view that reality can be best understood by dividing it into its smallest parts and examining them. All models seem reductionistic, in part, because they involve analysis, and analysis involves breaking down material into component parts. Reductionism assumes that the parts (of a model or system) exist independently, and that all complex phenomena can be reduced to independent parts. "But not every attempt to bring order or simplicity to a situation is a reduction: reduction involves a relation between levels. In a reduction, phenomena on one level or sublevel are explained in terms of realities on what is deemed a more basic or sublevel. Without this interlevel and explanatory relationship, there is no reduction" (Jones, 2000, p. 21). So, judgments about reductionism should consider whether a hierarchical structure is involved. In medicine, for example, a variety of systems can be reduced to hierarchical levels and parts. As pragmatic as this approach may be, reductionism comes at a cost: loss of the big picture. Perhaps the popularity of complementary and alternative medicine can be explained by a need for a holistic, or less reductionistic, approach to health care.

Another consideration is the origin of ethical models. Most ethical models and codes originate from an authority: a well-known theory, a professional organization, or an expert. These models and codes are deductive (top down); they follow an authoritative set of rules or principles. Other codes, such as the current Statement of Values and Ethics of the Midwives Alliance of North America (MANA), stem from membership input (A. Frye, personal communication, July 15, 2009). Similar to contextual theories, they are inductive (bottom up), originating from the grassroots of an organization.

Rather than a deductive or inductive model, Beauchamp and Childress (2009) propose a "reflective equilibrium" model whereby conflicts between moral theory and considered judgments require continual adjustments to maintain equilibrium. In other words, applied ethics requires an ability to apply *moral theory* to *contextual ethical thinking* through critical evaluation of both in an effort to make these two compatible. "Equilibrium occurs after one evaluates the strengths and weaknesses of all plausible moral judgments, principles, and relevant background theories, incorporating as wide a variety of kinds and levels of legitimate beliefs as possible," including particular cases (Beauchamp & Childress, 2009, p. 383). In this way, contextual data that influence our moral outlook can be weighed with moral theory in a way that aligns with the practitioner's own experience of the situation. A conscientious practitioner must also consider that what sits well with her may not be in the client's best interest. Reflective equilibrium is a way to look at ethical thinking as ever-evolving and informed by a multitude of influences

To address the gap in understanding how principles and codes make sense in the context of daily practice, we present a new model for midwives, the Midwives' Ecosystemic Model of Ethical Thinking (MEMET), that focuses on ethical thinking rather than decision making, because ethics is a set of skills and, we argue, a morality of care.

THEORETICAL EXPLANATION FOR THE MIDWIVES' ECOSYSTEMIC MODEL OF ETHICAL THINKING

Midwives use ethics in daily practice, operating on the knowledge and experience that they have gained while working within interrelated contexts. We have labeled these contexts in an effort to understand how they influence our ethical thinking. They include the supportive network, practice setting, cultural milieu, and historical place and time. At the center of this process is the midwife-client relationship, a reflection of the Midwives Model of Care (MMOC) (Rothman, 1979) and individual factors that the midwife and client each bring to the relationship. In this model of ethical thinking, ethical principles are mere abstractions unless the midwife has mastered their meaning and use within the context of her work.

We begin the introduction to our ethical thinking model, the MEMET, by considering some of the influences that informed its creation. Our collective educational backgrounds include psychology, gender studies, feminist critical thinking, midwifery, and applied ethics. These disciplines have informed our worldview and led to our shared understanding of ethical thinking for midwives. We have researched the literature abroad for guidance in ethics for midwives, because there is a dearth of research on the topic in the United States. By synthesizing ecological models, feminist virtue ethics, moral developmental theory, deconstructivist approaches, systems theory, the MMOC, and the existing data on ethics in midwifery, we have proposed a model of ethical thinking. This model is a reflection of the processes by which, we believe, ethical thinking occurs in the context of midwifery practice.

Faye Thompson (2002) draws the conclusion that normative ethical theory and principles are inadequate for midwifery care because they focus on behavior rather than human relationships and practical applications. She explored women's and midwives' perspectives on ethics through interviews.

> The mothers and midwives generally considered that the ethical response from mainstream maternity service providers was inadequate when it derived from abstract theory, standardization and 'product-efficiency' philosophy, and when it rendered the individual woman invisible. Institutional approaches that seemed to use the universal principles . . . were ethically adequate for these mothers and midwives only if the practitioner also considered context, individual rights, virtues of personal character and relationship. (Thompson, 2003, p. 593)

Perceiving ethical situations as embedded in relationship and context mirrors the historic work of Carol Gilligan (1982), once a student of Lawrence Kohlberg and moral development. Kohlberg (1981) focused his research on data gathered from young men, validating a justice perspective of morality that is highly individualistic. One way that Kohlberg assessed moral reasoning was through the presentation of ethical dilemmas. For example,

> In Europe a woman was near death from a special kind of cancer. There was one drug that doctors thought might save her. It was a form of radium that a druggist

in the same town had recently discovered. The drug was expensive to make, but the druggist was charging ten times what the drug cost to make. He paid $200 for the radium and charged $2,000 for a small dose of the drug. The sick woman's husband, Heinz, went to everyone he knew to borrow the money, but he could only get together about $1,000, which is half of what it cost. He told the druggist that his wife was dying, and asked him to sell it cheaper or let him pay later. But the druggist said, "No, I discovered the drug and I'm going to make money on it." So Heinz got desperate and began to think about breaking into the man's store to steal the drug for his wife. Should Heinz steal the drug? (Kohlberg, 1963, p. 12)

Kohlberg was interested not only in each participant's answer to the question, but also, more important, the reasoning behind the answer. Based on the reasoning provided, Kohlberg determined the level of moral development of the participant. A major criticism of his ranking system of six stages is that it focuses on the individual to the exclusion of the context. For example, in Kohlberg's model, reasoning might take the form of obedience (follow the rule), self-interest (get what you want), or universal principles of justice (a human life is more valuable than money). His initial study consistently showed women scoring lower in moral development, and subsequent research using his scales showed nurses as a subset being morally deficient (Crisham, 1981, and Ketefian, 1987, as cited in Lützén, 1997).

Gilligan (1982), however, studying young women, found contrasting cognitive processes of moral judgment that originated within a caring perspective: "for the very traits that traditionally have defined the 'goodness' of women, their care for and sensitivity to the needs of others, are those that mark them as deficient in moral development" (p. 18). In short, women are not morally deficient, says Gilligan, but different in their ways of making moral decisions from what Kohlberg proposed.

In comparing Kohlberg and Gilligan, Lawrence Blum (1988) argues that Gilligan discovered a new territory for moral theory, outside the objective and subjective, the personal and the impersonal. She found that care in relationships is, in and of itself, important morally. Further, Blum finds logical reasoning to support Gilligan's position that principles alone are inadequate:

I want to argue that what it takes to bring such principles to bear on individual situations involves qualities of character and sensibilities which are themselves moral and which go beyond the straightforward process of consulting a principle and then conforming one's will and action to it. Specifically I will argue that knowing that the particular situation which the agent is facing is one which calls for the particular principle in question and knowing how to apply the principle in question are capacities which, in the domain of personal relations (and perhaps elsewhere too), are intimately connected with care for individual persons. Such particularized,

> caring understanding is integral to an adequate meeting of the agent's moral responsibilities and cannot be generated from universal principle alone. (Blum, 1988, p. 485)

Thus, caring is an important moral quality that is inherent in effectively applying ethical principles. We believe that care is integral to the midwife-client relationship. The MMOC facilitates the midwife-client relationship, and the morality of caring is embedded within that relationship. When midwives apply ethical principles, they do so with compassionate caring. Ethical thinking occurs within a context of care that involves women and their relationship with caregivers. Next, we consider ethical thinking in the larger context of midwifery practice.

We also draw upon systems theory (Capra, 1996) in describing the nature of midwifery care. A human system, such as a family, a school, or a business, is composed of individuals. However, a basic premise of systems theory holds that the whole is greater than the sum of its parts. For example, a family system is more than the individuals who compose it; the system also includes the relationships, interactions, and connections between and across members. Moreover, systems theory recognizes ways in which changes to one part of a system affect all other parts. Consider how a new baby does not merely increase a family size by one, but also affects the parents, siblings, parent-child relationships, and parent-parent relationship. Moreover, impact is bidirectional, which is to say that each member of the system affects and is affected by each other member. Trying to understand one part of a system by isolating it fails to take into consideration the ways in which that part functions in real life. A systems approach suggests that the parts can only truly be understood in the context of the whole. For example, a child's behavioral challenges are best understood in the context of the family system. Additionally, the parts of the system are interdependent. Systems theory has great potential and applicability for midwifery and ethical decision making. Midwives view mother-baby units as systems, understand the role of pregnancy and childbirth in the client's family system, and even become a part of a system of care. Rather than occurring individually by the midwife or client, ethical thinking occurs in the space between the aforementioned individuals, within the clinical relationship.

Conceptually, the Ecological Model of Development best situates midwives' ethical thinking within an ecological context. The first ecological model was designed by Urie Bronfenbrenner (1979) to place human development within a holistic context of influences, including immediate influences (e.g., family, school) and larger systems of influence (e.g., community and culture). Standing in sharp contrast to prior models of development, Bronfenbrenner's approach views the individual as an active participant in his growth and development.

Moreover, the individual is affected by and affects the environmental systems in which he develops. As such, a child is shaped by her family, just as she in turn shapes the family. Additionally, she is affected by cultural, social, and political phenomena that are far removed from her immediate surroundings (e.g., health-care policy reform). As Bronfenbrenner explains,

> [L]ying at the very core of an ecological orientation and distinguishing it most sharply from prevailing approaches to the study of human development is the concern with the progressive accommodation between a growing human organism and its immediate environment, *and* the way in which this relation is mediated by forces emanating from more remote regions in the larger physical and social milieu. The ecology of human development lies at a point of convergence among the disciplines of the biological, psychological, and social sciences and they bear on the evolution of the individual in society. (p. 13)

Because individuals are intertwined with their ecological systems, any effort to understand the individual isolated from his or her environment falls short of a comprehensive analysis. With an authentic approach, "the properties of the person and of the environment, the structure of environmental settings, and the processes taking place within and between them must be viewed as interdependent and analyzed in systems terms" (Bronfenbrenner, 1979, p. 41). Earlier in this chapter we defined and discussed systems theory.

Bronfenbrenner's (1979) ecological perspective can be found in models designed specifically for explaining health and health care. Other models have been used as conceptual tools that assist understanding broad influences on human health, including social and economic influences. These models illustrate hierarchies that determine health and the strategies to integrate policies, because the influences in one area of the model affect the whole (Hancock, 1993). This is in contrast to reductionism, in which systems are broken down into independent parts.

We value ecological perspectives in the context of ethical decision making for midwifery because these models resonate with the context of midwifery care: midwives and clients working as a system, integrating family and community, with a keen awareness of cultural, social, and political influences. As we introduce and explain our model of ethical decision making in this chapter, the ecological perspective will emerge as a helpful way of putting compassionate care and ethics into the complexity of real life practice.

When midwives think about ethics in their daily practice and apply ethical reasoning in meaningful ways that serve women within the midwife-client relationship, they are "doing ethics." We borrow this concept from the field of gender studies. In the late 1980s, gender scholars began to conceptualize gender as social/psychological behaviors and cognitions in which people actively engage through acting and enforcing gender roles. "Doing gender" assisted researchers in looking at gender in new and critical ways by transforming the noun *gender* into a verb, illustrating how people use gender (as you would use any other tool) in their daily lives. "An understanding of how gender is produced in social situations will afford clarification of the interactional scaffolding of social structure and the social control processes that sustain it" (West & Zimmerman, 1987, p. 147). By placing ethics in a similar light, we (midwives) become empowered participants in ethical thinking and acting. To accurately analyze the ways that midwives "do ethics," we acknowledge the embedded nature of ethical thinking and decision making and how midwives apply knowledge of ethics within care contexts.

What follows is a description of our proposed MEMET model (Figure 12-1) that illustrates how midwives think and make decisions about (i.e., "do") ethics. The model encompasses theories that we have discussed in this chapter from

---

Figure 12-1   Ecosystemic model of ethical thinking in midwifery.

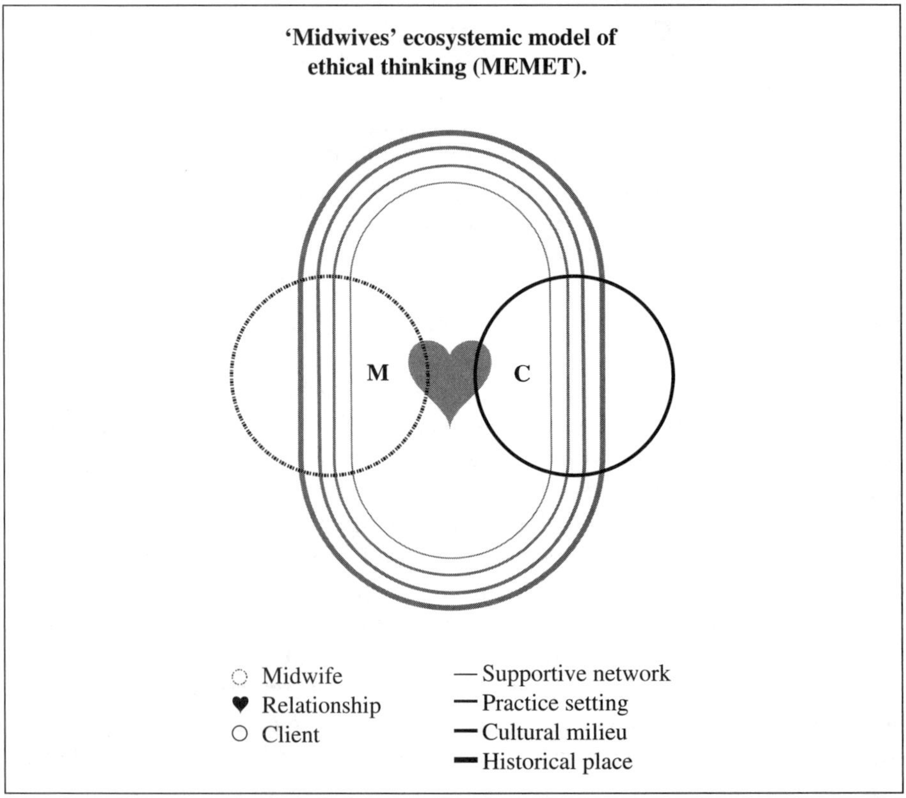

'Midwives' ecosystemic model of
ethical thinking (MEMET).

M   C

○ Midwife   — Supportive network
♥ Relationship   — Practice setting
○ Client   — Cultural milieu
                     ▬ Historical place

gender studies, moral development, and human ecology. The model is further informed by the research of Faye Thompson (2002, 2003, 2004) and feminist virtue ethics. We believe that it captures the MMOC and balances contextual ethics with ethical codes and principles, while striving to reach the equilibrium described by Beauchamp and Childress (2009), whereby ethical thinking is ever evolving and informed by a multitude of influences.

Midwife-Client Relationship

We begin our discussion of our model at the center of midwifery care: the midwife-client relationship. In doing so, we must first identify the client (see Chapter 5). The intertwined nature of pregnancy informs our definition of "client" as including the mother and her fetus. Other client definitions may include the mother's partner or her other family members, or all of these. The client is the person or persons with whom the midwife's primary responsibilities lie. Consider the client definition as we discuss the midwife-client relationship.

Rather than being an elite expert, midwives typically relate to mothers as a "professional friend" (Thompson, 2003, 2004). This is the crux of the MMOC: being "with woman," where the woman is the primary decision maker and an active partner in her health care. This contrasts with the physician-patient relationship (Rooks, 1999). At the heart of the midwifery model is caring. Some may regard the "professional friend" status as ethically problematic, given concerns about multiple relationships and objectivity (see Chapter 6). Midwives must consider the difference between being friends with clients and being "professional friends."

Perhaps this concept of professional friend is best illustrated by the ethic of care, in accordance with Blum's (1988) analysis of Carol Gilligan's work. Joyce Thompson (2007) defines the ethic of care as having three components: compassion, fidelity, and competence. She elaborates, "If you truly care about another person, you will always remain competent in your midwifery practice . . . you will be compassionate in your interactions . . . [and] faithful in the relationship, going beyond the legal aspect of contract to the ethical aspects of covenant fidelity" (p. 284). Herein lies the responsibility of the midwife: the professional friend has an ethical obligation to care.

Both the client and the midwife bring unique qualities to the relationship. A midwife's prior knowledge and experience, her scope of practice, communication style, and orientation, or how she views her role as the midwife (Thompson 2003), all factor into the relationship. Similarly, the client's own communication style, her choices regarding her care, and her own cognitive facilities and sense of responsibility inform the midwife-client relationship. Other personal characteristics, such as socioeconomic status, ethnicity, education level, marital status, and age may inform the midwife-client relationship. We will call these *midwife characteristics* and *client characteristics*, respectively.

Shared characteristics in the midwife-client relationship, such as a sense of partnership, trust, and intimacy, further factor into the equation. A relationship that is built on trust and mutual respect will positively inform ethical thinking within that relationship. As implied in the Ecological Model of Human Development (Bronfenbrenner, 1979) and systems theory (Capra, 1996), some factors coexist within individuals and outside them. For example, a distrustful person may also be involved in relationships that are devoid of trust. In midwifery practice, the midwife may confront an ethical dilemma, but the dilemma also persists in her relationship with her client and in the larger context of her practice or culture.

Whereas some ethical dilemmas originate in the midwife-client relationship (e.g., a midwife fails to obtain informed consent), others may originate from the practice setting (e.g., hospital policy requires a midwife to act in violation of her ethics) or elsewhere. Regardless, the immediate need of the client and the nature of the ethical dilemma have direct bearing on each person in the relationship and their collective approach to ethical problem solving. The influence of both is stronger within the relationship than in contexts outside the relationship. For example, the mother's state of anemia (need of the client) has more immediate bearing on the midwife and the client than on the lab where the blood was analyzed. Also, a breach of confidentiality of her lab results (nature of the ethical dilemma) places more tension on the midwife-client relationship than on other spheres of influence. This is because ethical decisions are typically made within the clinical relationship. The ethical burden lies within the relationship, so the ethical dilemma will be highly salient within that relationship. Exceptions to this rule include cases where ethical dilemmas originate outside the clinical relationship *and* do not directly affect the midwife-client relationship. For example, bullying in midwife-to-midwife relationships rarely directly affects the individual client, although bullying in midwifery may affect a midwife's practice in general, and have an overall negative impact on the profession.

As we explore other levels of the model, keep in mind the emphasis on the midwife-client relationship. It is important to describe the contexts in which midwives and clients operate in order to adequately understand ethical thinking and decision making. We begin doing this by exploring the influences that have direct impact on the midwife-client relationship.

Supportive Network

The first intervening sphere of influence includes the immediate supportive network: other care providers, family, and friends. These are other people to whom the midwife and client have a personal responsibility, but they are not the midwife's primary responsibility. Remember, it is the client to whom the midwife has primary responsibility. The individuals in this level of influence have direct bearing on the midwife-client relationship, and vice versa. They exist in the immediate environment, and may include the client's partner, the client's mother, the client's other children, nurses, midwife partners, and physicians.

The supportive network may involve many different types of influences, including *positive elements*, such as a good friend who believes in the woman's choices and supports them fully. *Conflicting elements* may include another care provider who does not support the woman's choices or who does not accept the midwife's role. When midwives and clients make ethical decisions, the supportive network (of both conflicting and positive elements) can challenge or affirm their process.

The nature of this collective influence may, in turn, affect the midwife's actions and her relationship with the client (i.e., ethical decisions). We conceptualize this by use of systems theory. The clinical relationship and the supportive network both influence and are influenced by one another. In turn, all aspects of the system are engaged, akin to Bronfenbrenner's (1979) Ecological Model of Human Development. For example, a midwife and client will usually consider a collaborating doctor's opinion when making a decision. The decision that is made is likely to have an impact on the physician and other aspects of the supportive network, including nurses and the client's family members. However, the supportive network is not only affected by the clinical relationship but also by other realms of influence, including the practice setting.

Practice Setting

The practice setting includes physical, organizational, social, and political structures. Like the supportive network, there are both positive and conflicting elements in the practice setting. Elements of the practice setting have bidirectional influences on one another, as well as on other contextual layers of the MEMET, including the midwife-client relationship.

A midwife's office space may be situated in a practice with an obstetrician. This physical setting may influence the midwife-client relationship in several possible ways, including length of appointments, the presence of nursing and office staff, the physical décor, and perhaps even the midwife's own orientation (how she sees her role as a midwife). Imagine that the midwife would much prefer a cozy office space, with comfortable seating for her clients, whereas her actual office space is set up with an examination table, a single hard-backed chair, and a swivel stool for the provider. This midwife would, perhaps, also prefer 30-minute prenatal appointments, but is bound by office policy to limit routine appointments to 15 minutes. These structures, both physical and organizational, are likely to affect both the supportive network (the client's partner and children, for example, who do not attend prenatal appointments because of lack of space) and the midwife-client relationship (which becomes more of a clinical relationship than that of a personal friend who sits down and serves tea). Likewise, the supportive network (such as the obstetrician who shares office space with the midwife) affects both the practice setting (by imposing a more clinical feeling in the office) and the midwife-client relationship (by imposing strict time limits on appointments).

If a midwife is practicing in a hospital, the midwife-client relationship is informed by the midwife's role as defined by hospital policy and politics, both formally and informally. The power structure at the hospital may include the midwife as an autonomous primary care provider, or the hospital may have a hierarchical structure in which the midwife operates under close supervision by a physician or another midwife. The power that the midwife has within the context of the organization in which she works will greatly define her relationship with her clients. The midwife and client may also affect this practice setting. If a subordinate midwife supports a client's decision to refuse an induction scheduled for the 41st week of pregnancy, this decision may have a wide range of influences on the practice setting, including hospital policy, politics, and organization.

Midwives who practice in out-of-hospital settings are likely to have less tension in their practice settings, because they are usually working with greater autonomy and have more control over their work environment. Many birth center and homebirth midwives write their own protocols, for example. Yet, practice setting is still a contextual layer that influences the midwife-client relationship and informs midwives' ethical decision making. Birth centers are regulated by governing agencies that often restrict scope of practice in ways that are uncommon in homebirth settings, and birth center midwives often share being on call. In contrast, a homebirth midwife is likely to be on call for her clients 24 hours a day. These characteristics of practice setting are among numerous others that affect ethical thinking for midwives.

When midwives utilize the MMOC, midwifery care is woman centered, in contrast to the policies and politics of many practice settings. Thus, the practice setting is a likely source of tension on the midwife-client relationship. As illustrated by our model of ethical thinking, both the client and midwife are influenced by the practice setting. This influence exerts an impact on the midwife-client relationship, which, in turn, affects the practice setting. The practice setting is often a reflection of the larger cultural context.

Cultural Milieu

Milieu is a French word meaning the setting in which something develops. The cultural milieu is a soup of powerful influences that are not typically directly linked to the midwife-client relationship. These influences may be community based or related to issues of legal jurisdiction and standards of care, and shape the role of midwives. Professional organizations, including local, state, and national associations, often define standards of practice and codes that create social expectations. These and other informal community standards that evolve over time permeate the practice setting as well as the midwife-client relationship.

Midwives often deal with issues related to the cultural milieu, especially if they work in out-of-hospital practice settings. When a homebirth midwife transports a client to the hospital, she often experiences dissonance, because her role there is largely defined by state or local jurisdictions, as well as hospital policy (practice setting). Initially the primary caregiver, the midwife usually transfers the care of her client to a physician and team of nurses. This process may go very smoothly if the midwife has a professional relationship with the physicians and staff at the hospital, if her community recognizes her role in maternity care, and if she is legally licensed to practice. One can imagine the difficulties that the midwife and client may encounter if home birth is illegal in their state, if physicians do not allow the midwife to accompany her client, or if the medical community does not comprehend the midwife's role. All of this affects her relationship with her client as well as her ethical decision making.

The cultural milieu, in the form of regulatory boards, standards of practice, laws, and ethical codes, influences midwives' ethical thinking. Although they know that these systems exist, midwives and clients may not always be aware of their influence. Just as a fish is unaware of the water in which it swims, most people are unaware of the subtle and implicit social structures of the systems in which they operate. Our model encourages midwives to look at the structures that they may rarely notice, and consider how they affect ethical thinking. Sandra Bem (1993) writes about social constructivism and how it allows one to see the lens through which one typically views the world. This allows a critical thinker to examine assumptions, protocols, and other systematic processes with some level of objectivity. Although we can never completely step outside our own worlds of influence and examine them objectively, we can acknowledge that these structures exist and try to understand them.

As abstract as it may seem, the cultural milieu is an ever-present influence on ethical thinking. Midwives' scope of practice, codes of conduct and ethics, and standards of care are defined by the cultural milieu, and it is compelling to consider how the cultural milieu, in turn, relates to our practice setting, our supportive network, and our relationships with clients. For example, if a midwife is practicing under state laws that restrict her access to potentially life-saving medications, she may be ethically driven to break the law in order to provide safe maternity care. To do otherwise may put her client at great risk. Yet, by breaking the law, the midwife may inadvertently attract grievances upon her practice. The cultural milieu largely reflects the historical place in which it is situated.

Historical Place

Historical place is an umbrella term to summarize broad cultural belief systems, including religion, philosophy, and values. It includes economic systems that are reflected in the rising cost of health care and inaccessibility to education and other services for segments of the population. It encompasses societal attitudes regarding class, ethnicity, and gender that influence every other context in which we practice. It is the stock of the soup recipe. It may also be conceptualized as the space through which our model moves.

The historical place includes aspects of technology that permeate our communities and standards of care (cultural milieu), as well as our physical and organizational structures (practice setting), our coworkers (supportive network), and our client relationships. Technology has a huge impact on contemporary midwifery practice. Technological intervention in childbirth has been a mainstay of modern medicine. Because the MMOC includes a minimization of technological interventions, midwives often struggle with that aspect of historical place. Obvious examples include external fetal monitoring, epidurals, induction, and amniocentesis. Midwives who interface the most with the medical model are more likely to encounter technological birth (i.e., the technocratic model described by Robbie Davis-Floyd, 2004).

Historical place also includes aspects of contemporary society that are salient to midwifery care and ethics. The current dominant perceptions of childbirth as a painful experience that one must endure to attain children, an experience that it is advisable to attempt to separate from by use of anesthesia; as an institutionalized experience, rather than a private one; and as a medical event, rather than a developmental one, are historical social constructs that change according to the times and reflect struggles for power. According to Foucault (1978), these social constructs inform our culture and care models. Williams (1997) affirms an ecological systemic approach as she expands on Foucault:

> He stresses that it is the understanding of the mechanisms of power that is important and suggests looking at its effects by focusing on opposition struggles at the periphery and then tracing inwards. This helps to move away from the single concept of domination towards a notion of the circulating network of power existing at different levels and in different forms throughout society. In trying to regain control of childbirth, women have access to certain forms of power but are also simultaneously influenced by it. The same is true for the obstetrician and midwife. (p. 233)

Historical place is another lens through which we view our world. When we look at broad cultural constructs related to childbirth, mothering, and the place of midwives in this process, we begin to understand the power struggles that have dominated midwifery: between obstetricians and midwives, between certified nurse–midwives and certified professional midwives, and the power struggles and bullying that occur among individual midwives. Midwives serve women and their families within a culture that largely does not value their work. Therefore, midwives may seek power in their profession by differentiating themselves from other midwives and imposing hierarchical structures that reinforce divisions. To bring the midwife-client relationship to the center of this discussion, as it is centrally located in the MEMET, one must consider how midwives and women experience the historical place in their clinical relationships. The MEMET may be used as both a descriptive tool and, in this case, an analytical one.

ANALYSIS OF THE MODEL

The MEMET has a number of possible functions. As a descriptive tool, it illustrates midwives' relationship-centered caring perspective in making ethical decisions. Scholars and midwives may consider its validity in explaining ethical thinking for midwives. It is hoped this will generate further research. Our goal is to present it as a viable model, the validity of which is to be determined over time. "External validity is the degree to which the conclusions in your study would hold for other persons in other places and at other times" (Trochim, 2006, n.p.). For now we can only consider its validity externally by comparison with other models and research findings.

In the space we have here, we limit our analysis of validity to the most widely published model of ethical decision making for midwives. Aspects of the Thompson and Thompson Bioethical Decision-Making Model (Table 12-1; Thompson, 2007) support the validity of the MEMET, especially the first four steps of their model. In the first step, key individuals are considered. These relate to both the MEMET's *supportive network* and *practice setting*. Institutional policies, which relate to both *practice setting* and *cultural milieu*, are measured, along with legal constraints, in the second step. Step 3 relates to the MEMET's *cultural milieu* and *historical place*: "explore historical roots" and "discuss societal/cultural views" of each issue. Further, step 4 seems to underline the nature of subjective influence when it instructs the clinician to "understand personal values affected by situation/ethical issues raised." In this step, Thompson and Thompson recognize that the practitioner has a personal reaction to ethical dilemmas, but they do not expand on this notion. The MEMET adds dimension to this concept, identifying influences both within and outside the individual that affect ethical thinking. These facets of the Thompson and Thompson model support the validity of the MEMET.

Earlier in the chapter, we included theoretical support for the MEMET, including gender studies, systems theory, and theories of moral and ecological development. Although these have stimulated a good deal of research in various disciplines, their use here is novel. Their applicability in the context of ethical thinking for midwives will be assessed over time. The research that we have covered in this text on midwifery and biomedical ethics has informed the model, and we have taken steps to include relevant research in its construction. Another way to measure the validity of a model is to examine its utility.

The MEMET has practical uses. For analysis, the MEMET allows the individual midwife to consider her own ethical dilemma in light of the MMOC and other powerful environmental influences. In this regard, the MEMET offers something novel, set apart from other ethical models to date. In terms of application, the MEMET may be used alongside bioethical decision-making models when grappling with ethical dilemmas. Decision-making models are successful in providing step-by-step guidance in addressing problems, but they generally lack explanation of contextual factors that influence a midwife's decision-making process. Independently, the MEMET serves as a guide to midwives, where they can situate their approach to ethical dilemmas. Rather than taking a principle-based approach to ethics without regard for relational ties, or a purely contextual approach in which ethics are relative, the MEMET balances the need for the midwife to both care and think critically when confronted with ethical dilemmas.

Teaching ethical thinking is an important function of the model. As midwives apply ethical principles, they are instructed to do so within the midwife-client relationship. One may choose a topic within this text and think about the concept within the MEMET. "How should a midwife approach informed consent?" and other such queries can be answered by use of this model. By referring to case examples, teachers and preceptors can situate ethical thinking into the MMOC by use of the MEMET. Teaching midwives to think ethically is essential to ethical practice (Alison Bastien, personal communication, August 7, 2009).

The MEMET may be used during peer reviews to reflect on ethical thinking in case studies and related ethical discourse. Further use of the MEMET at conferences and ethics training sessions is likely to spark debate and further research. These efforts will further advance our understanding of midwifery ethics.

To this end, midwifery practice may be brought home and held to midwifery standards. As pregnancy and childbirth have become medicalized, midwives have developed professionally out of necessity and a desire to collaborate with other healthcare professionals. Professionalization has often led to adoption of medical standards of care and ethics. There is much to be learned by studying medical ethics. In this book, we have chosen to focus on applied ethics for its practicality, yet we did not dispense with bioethical principles. As midwives use our book and model in their practice, we hope they will find ethical equilibrium by considering both principles and context (Beauchamp & Childress, 2009) and that they will use a morality of care (Gilligan, 1982).

CASE EXAMPLES

CASE 1

Sue Ellen meets Jovita after the latter recently moved from Mexico City. Sue Ellen works at a large hospital unit in New York City. Jovita had already had three other babies vaginally with a Mexican physician attending. She had an episiotomy at each birth. Sue Ellen explains to Jovita that episiotomies are not the standard of care in her community and are considered to be largely unnecessary and potentially harmful. Jovita is adamant that she desires an episiotomy and believes that it will protect her vagina, rectum, and pelvic floor from a dysfunction that she has heard about from her elders.

Questions

1. How does this case fit into the MEMET?
2. Which key ethical standards and codes should Sue Ellen consider and discuss with her client?
3. How does an ethic of care relate to this case?

Analysis

The relationship between Jovita and her midwife, Sue Ellen, is just in its infancy. They have a range of issues to bridge between them, not the least of which is cultural. In making ethical decisions, the midwife considers her clinical relationship as well as the other contextual factors that are relevant. A number of contextual issues are salient to this case. We will use the structure of the MEMET to examine each.

Let's begin at the center of the model: the clinical relationship. The midwife's own characteristics, as well as the client's, factor into the clinical relationship. Jovita is an immigrant, and she clearly has some cultural views regarding episiotomy. The midwife's characteristics will include her scope of practice (Does she do episiotomies?), her training (Are episiotomies ever done electively?), and her cultural competency (see Chapter 10). Depending on Sue Ellen's orientation (how she sees her role as midwife), she may approach this situation collabora-tively or authoritatively. If she identifies strongly with the MMOC, she will likely seek a collaborative solution to the dilemma.

Further influences on ethical thinking in this case can be found in the con-textual layers of the model. The supportive network may include such factors as the client's familial support. If influential members of her family advise her to seek an episiotomy, they are relevant to this dilemma. Similarly, if the midwife has a professional partner who may be involved in the birth, she or he is also part of that supportive network that warrants consideration in this case.

Moving outward from the center, the next contextual layer is the practice set-ting. Inclusive are hospital policies regarding episiotomies, as well as political support for episiotomy as an elective procedure. The midwife may be bound by certain protocols related to episiotomies that inform her practice.

The contextual layers of cultural milieu and historical place usually have in-direct influence on the clinical relationship, but they are influential factors in this case. Standards of care, community values, and legal considerations usually fall within the cultural milieu. Whether it is atypical for a midwife to perform an episiotomy or if it is commonplace, the standards of care within a community heavily inform a midwife's practice and ethical thinking. Likewise, other com-munity values and legal considerations regarding episiotomy are involved. More broadly, historical place may affect the availability of episiotomy, and current views regarding childbirth may relate to the midwife's views as well. She may see episiotomy as part of the medicalization of birth that women seek (as part of their participation in the historical place) in a technological society. Both midwife's and client's views and experiences are shaped by the cultural milieu and his-torical place, and these affect the ethical thinking that occurs within their rela-tionship and the practice settings and support networks in which they live and work.

If Sue Ellen is conscientious of the above influences, she may also be aware of some of the ethical standards and codes that relate to her client's request. These have to do with principles of diversity, autonomy, and nonmaleficence. First, she can consider the diversity factor, because it is in the forefront of her relationship with Jovita. The code of ethics of the American College of Nurse Midwives (ACNM, 2008) says that midwives will act without discrimination and will work within their own level of cultural competency. As explained in Chap-ter 10, cultural competence involves respecting cultural difference while mini-mizing negative consequences associated with cultural differences. The International Confederation of Midwives (ICM, 2003) states that midwives re-spect cultural diversity and work to eliminate harmful cultural practices. A sec-ond ethical standard, which relates to autonomy, is informed choice. ACNM and ICM both maintain a woman's right to informed consent and acceptance of responsibility for the outcomes related to her choices. A midwife in Sue Ellen's position is likely to approach Jovita's request by educating her about the risks and benefits of episiotomy, as well as the alternatives. Finally, a midwife's responsibility to do no harm to her client (see Chapter 1) will contribute to her ethical thinking and actions.

The ethics of care involve compassion, competency, and loyalty. These are all aspects of the professional friend. Morality from a caring perspective involves thinking not only about the other (the client), but also about oneself. A midwife may choose to refer a client to another care provider if she believes that performing an episiotomy at a normal birth is potentially harmful to the woman and the midwife's own sense of ethics. This is not the only possible outcome from a caring perspective. A different midwife might consider the woman's cultural meanings and choices to be the most defining characteristic of protecting the client's autonomy and honoring her culture. She may agree to the episiotomy on those ethical grounds. A third midwife might take a different approach, one of paternalism, and refuse to do the episiotomy without referring to another provider. This is another possible outcome, but not one that we endorse. However, if the midwife and client come to a mutual agreement, such that both the client's and the midwife's dignity is maintained, then a midwife's refusal to perform an episiotomy may be appropriate and reflect the ethics of care.

CASE 2

Lizzy is a midwife with 20 years of experience; much of her career was spent working under the supervision of physicians at a small rural hospital in the Midwest. She embarks on a new practice setting after home birth becomes legal in her state. Years ago, she had birthed her own children at home with a direct-entry midwife (DEM), and she wants to serve childbearing women in this capacity. She contacts some of the midwives who practiced under the radar for years when the old law against home birth was enforced. Now these midwives are licensed. Carlene, a licensed homebirth midwife, agrees to allow Lizzy to attend home births with her. Once she leaves the hospital, Lizzy is no longer covered by malpractice insurance by her supervising physician. Lizzy is accustomed to having malpractice insurance coverage, and wants Carlene to cover her in exchange for her services at births. Carlene adamantly opposes malpractice insurance for midwives, and feels that it is the best way to ensure one will be sued. Her position is that midwives do not practice medicine and are not covered by most insurance companies; the ones that will cover midwives are too expensive for most private practices.

Questions

1. In the MEMET, what influences are salient to Lizzy's dilemma?
2. How can Lizzy use applied ethics and other tools to solve her dilemma?
3. Is Lizzy ethically obligated to carry malpractice insurance to practice midwifery?

Analysis

Although it is unclear whether Lizzy has any current homebirth clients, we can still situate her ethical dilemma in relation to her (past, present, or future) clients. Although the model was not intended to cover the entire scope of ethical problems in the field of midwifery, it can be applied to many that are not obviously centered on the clinical relationship. Lizzy's primary responsibility is to her clients, whether they are currently in her care or not. Let's first consider the ramifications of malpractice insurance on the client. The following questions are pertinent: Can the client be harmed by Lizzy's insurance coverage status? Is Lizzy's relationship with her client likely to be negatively affected by carrying or not carrying insurance? In considering how to solve this ethical dilemma, Lizzy may benefit from considering the clinical relationship. She may also be informed by considering the other contextual layers in the model.

For this situation, it may be difficult to predict how clients' family members and other providers who collaborate on care (the supportive network) may influence the malpractice insurance dilemma. Does the practice setting affect Lizzy's ethical dilemma regarding malpractice insurance? If most homebirth midwives do not carry insurance, and it is not available or affordable, then there is little pressure from the practice setting to purchase insurance. Lizzy may want to consider other factors within the cultural milieu, such as the standard of care and the role of homebirth midwives in her community. She may find that although homebirth midwives are not insured, the general public in her area expects healthcare providers to carry insurance. Her analysis of these cultural findings will affect her ethical decision-making process. The final contextual layer to consider is historical place. National trends across most industries are highly litigious, and the healthcare industry is perhaps the most litigious of them all, with obstetrics bearing the greatest burden of malpractice lawsuits. Lizzy may be fearful of lawsuits and uncomfortable practicing without malpractice insurance. A decision to carry insurance would most likely benefit her practice (especially in the case of an unfortunate outcome), rather than her clients. But one may argue that protecting a midwifery practice is protecting the choice of home birth for all future clients as well.

In our own analysis, we are unable to find any ethical standard or code that requires malpractice insurance. Additional guidance for this dilemma may be found by using a bioethical decision-making model, such as that of Thompson and Thompson (Thompson, 2007).

CASE 3

Donald is a midwife working in a suburban hospital on the East Coast. His client, Louise, desires a vaginal birth after cesarean (V-BAC). She meets all the characteristics of a good V-BAC candidate and is well prepared for the birth. She has hired a doula and has attended childbirth classes from a reputable instructor. Over the course of the pregnancy, Donald thoroughly explains the risks and benefits of a V-BAC to his client, while simultaneously preparing her for the possibility that a second surgical birth might be necessary.

When Louise begins labor spontaneously, Donald advises her to stay home with her doula until she is in an active labor phase. Donald meets Louise at the hospital, and Louise is 4 cm dilated with a strong labor pattern. The head of the labor and delivery unit is present when Louise is admitted, and he approaches Donald about the planned V-BAC. He doesn't support V-BACs, and although there is nothing explicitly stated in hospital policy against them, he insists that they are highly unusual there. He questions Donald's judgment in supporting his client's choice, and makes it clear to Donald that the slightest variation from normal in the client's labor progress will necessitate a surgical delivery.

Questions

1. How does this ethical dilemma fit in the framework of the MEMET?
2. How does it help Donald and Louise to think about the ethical dilemma in this way?
3. In what ways are the ethics of care inherent in this case?

Analysis

Donald and Louise have built a trusting relationship over the course of care that is based on mutual respect and good communication. Their relationship reflects the MMOC, which involves protecting a woman's autonomy and woman-centered control (Simonds, Rothman, & Meltzer Norman, 2006). Donald's first allegiance is to his client. This brings us to the MEMET, for the midwife-client relationship exists within a larger social context. Donald's experience with the head of the labor and delivery unit demonstrates the pressure that practice setting can place on the midwife-client relationship. Yet, it is also possible that the strength of said relationship may place tension on the practice setting in such a way that the organization responds. The bidirectional nature of the influences of one part of the model on the others is important to acknowledge. Doing so may help Donald understand that he is part of a larger system that is constantly in flux, rather than being a victim of a technologically and litigiously driven maternity system.

Because Louise hired a doula, it is likely that she, too, will play a role in the birth. The midwife may use the MEMET to understand that the doula's role bears direct influence on the client and the midwife-client relationship. Although Donald does not have primary responsibility for the doula, he must acknowledge her input because the client assigned her to that role. Other healthcare providers who may become directly involved with Louise's care will have similar influence.

Placing the dynamics of the supportive network and the practice setting within a broader framework, including cultural milieu and historical place, provides further opportunity for insights. If Donald is aware of the legal and political issues pertaining to his case, he may seek involvement in legislative efforts to expand the autonomy of his profession.

The MEMET may be instructional for Donald and provide him with greater awareness of the various contextual factors that he must weigh with ethical principles in his clinical relationship with Louise. This is where the ethics of care may collide with power structures that are inflexible and routine in their protocols.

REFERENCES

American College of Nurse-Midwives (ACNM). (2008). *American College of Nurse-Midwives code of ethics with explanatory statements*. Silver Spring, MD: Author.

Beauchamp, T. L., & Childress, J. F. (2009). *Principles of biomedical ethics* (6th ed.). New York: Oxford University Press.

Bem, S. L. (1993). *The lenses of gender: Transforming the debate on sexual inequality*. New Haven, CT: Yale University Press.

Blum, L. A. (1988). Gilligan and Kohlberg: Implications for moral theory. *Ethics, 98*(3), 472–491.

Bronfenbrenner, U. (1979). *The ecology of human development: Experiments by nature and design*. Cambridge, MA: Harvard University Press.

Capra, F. (1996). *The web of life: A new scientific understanding of living systems*. New York: Anchor Books.

Davis-Floyd, R. E. (2004). *Birth as an American rite of passage*. Berkeley, CA: University of California Press.

Foucault, M. (1978) *History of sexuality: Vol. 1. An introduction*. New York: Random House.

Gilligan, C. (1982). *In a different voice*. Cambridge, MA: Harvard University Press.

Hancock, T. (1993). Health, human development, and the community ecosystem: Three ecological models. *Health Promotion International, 8*(1), 41–47.

International Confederation of Midwives (ICM). (2003). *ICM international code of ethics for midwives*. Retrieved January 30, 2009, from http://www.internationalmidwives.org/Documentation/Coredocuments/tabid/322/Default.aspx

Jones, R. H. (2000). *Reductionism: Analysis and the fullness of reality*. Lewisburg, PA: Bucknell University Press.

Kohlberg, L. (1963). The development of children's orientations toward a moral order. *Vita Humana, 6*(1–2), 11–33.

Kohlberg, L. (1981). *The philosophy of moral development: Moral stages and the idea of justice*. San Francisco: Harper & Row.

Lützén, K. (1997). Nursing ethics into the next millennium: A context-sensitive approach for nursing ethics. *Nursing Ethics, 4*(3), 218–226.

Rooks, J. P. (1999). The midwifery model of care. *Journal of Nurse-Midwifery, 44*(4), 370–374.

Rothman, B. K. (1979). *Two models in maternity care: Defining and negotiating reality*. New York: New York University Press.

Simonds, W., Rothman, B. K., & Meltzer Norman, B. (2006). *Laboring on: Birth in transition in the United States*. New York: Routledge.

Thompson, F. E. (2002). Moving from codes of ethics to ethical relationships in midwifery practice. *Nursing Ethics, 9*(5), 522–536.

Thompson, F. E. (2003). The practice setting: Site of ethical conflict for some mothers and midwives. *Nursing Ethics, 10*(6), 588–601.

Thompson, F. E. (2004). *Mothers and midwives: The ethical journey*. London: Books for Midwives.

Thompson, J. E. (2007). Professional ethics. In L. A. Ament (Ed.), *Professional issues in midwifery* (pp. 277–300). Sudbury, MA: Jones and Bartlett.

Thompson, I. E., Melia, K. M., & Boyd, K. M. (2005). *Nursing ethics* (4th ed.). New York: Churchill Livingstone.

Trochim, W. M. K. (2006). External validity. *Research methods knowledge base*. Retrieved from http://www.socialresearchmethods.net/kb/external.php

Tschudin, V. (2003). *Ethics in nursing: The caring relationship*. London: Butterworth Heinemann.

West, C., & Zimmerman, D. H. (1987). Doing gender. *Gender and Society, 1*(2), 125–151.

Williams, J. (1997). The controlling power of childbirth in Britain. In H. Marland & A. M. Rafferty (Eds.), *Midwives, society and childbirth: Debates and controversies in the modern period* (pp. 232–248). London: Routledge.

The MANA Statement of Values and Ethics

We, as midwives, have a responsibility to educate ourselves and others regarding our values and ethics and to reflect them in our practices. Our exploration of ethical midwifery is a critical reflection of moral issues as they pertain to maternal and child health on every level. This statement is intended to provide guidance for professional conduct in the practice of midwifery, as well as for MANA's policy making, thereby promoting quality care for childbearing families. MANA recognizes this document as an open, ongoing articulation of our evolution regarding values and ethics.

We recognize that values often go unstated, and yet our ethics (how we act), proceed directly from a foundation of values. Since what we hold precious—that is, what we value—infuses and informs our ethical decisions and actions, the Midwives Alliance of North America wishes to explicitly affirm our values[1] as follows:

I. **Woman as an Individual with Unique Value and Worth**
    A. We value women and their creative, life-affirming and life-giving powers, which find expression in a diversity of ways.
    B. We value a woman's right to make choices regarding all aspects of her life.

II. **Mother and Baby as a Whole**
    A. We value the oneness of the pregnant mother and her unborn child, an inseparable and interdependent whole.
    B. We value the birth experience as a rite of passage; the sentient and sensitive nature of the newborn; and the right of each baby to be born in a caring and loving manner, without separation from mother and family.

---

[1]The membership largely agrees with the values that follow. However, some may word them differently or may leave out a few. This document is intended to prompt personal reflection and clarification, not to represent absolute opinions.

    C. We value the integrity of a woman's body and the right of each woman and baby to be totally supported in their efforts to achieve a natural, spontaneous vaginal birth.

    D. We value the breastfeeding relationship as the ideal way of nourishing and nurturing the newborn.

III. The Nature of Birth

    A. We value the essential mystery of birth.[2]

    B. We value pregnancy and birth as natural processes that technology will never supplant.[3]

    C. We value the integrity of life's experiences; the physical, emotional, mental, psychological and spiritual components of a process are inseparable.

    D. We value pregnancy and birth as personal, intimate, internal, sexual, and social events to be shared in the environment and with the attendants a woman chooses.[4]

    E. We value the learning experiences of life and birth.

    F. We value pregnancy and birth as processes that have lifelong impact on a woman's self-esteem, her health, her ability to nurture and her personal growth.

IV. The Art of Midwifery

    A. We value our right to practice the art of midwifery. We value our work as an ancient vocation of women that has existed as long as humans have lived on earth.

    B. We value expertise that incorporates academic knowledge, clinical skill, intuitive judgment and spiritual awareness.[5]

    C. We value all forms of midwifery education and acknowledge the ongoing wisdom of apprenticeship as the original model for training midwives.

    D. We value the art of nurturing the intrinsic normalcy of birth and recognize that each woman and baby have parameters of well-being unique to themselves.

    E. We value the empowerment of women in all aspects of life and particularly as their strength is realized during pregnancy, birth and the period

---

[2]Mystery is defined as something that has not or cannot be explained or understood; the quality or state of being incomprehensible or inexplicable; a tenet that cannot be understood in terms of human reason.

[3]Supplant means to supersede by force or cunning, to take the place of.

[4]In this context internal refers to birth happening within the body and psyche of the woman: ultimately she and only she can give birth.

[5]An expert is one whose knowledge and skill is specialized and profound, especially as the result of practical experience.

thereafter. We value the art of encouraging the open expression of that strength so women can birth unhindered and confident in their abilities and in our support.

F. We value skills that support a complicated pregnancy or birth to move toward a state of greater well-being or to be brought to the most healing conclusion possible. We value the art of letting go.[6]

G. We value the acceptance of death as a possible outcome of birth. We value our focus as supporting life rather than avoiding death.[7]

H. We value standing for what we believe in the face of social and political oppression.

V. **Woman as Mother**

A. We value a mother's intuitive knowledge of herself and her baby before, during and after birth.[8]

B. We value a woman's innate ability to nurture her pregnancy and birth her baby, the power and beauty of her body as it grows and the awesome strength summoned in labor.

C. We value the mother as the only direct care provider for her unborn child.[9]

D. We value supporting women in a nonjudgmental way, whatever their state of physical, emotional, social or spiritual health. We value the broadening of available resources whenever possible so that the desired goals of health, happiness and personal growth are realized according to a woman's needs and perceptions.

E. We value the right of each woman to choose a care giver appropriate to her needs and compatible with her belief system.

---

[6]This addresses our desire for an uncomplicated birth whenever possible and recognizes that there are times when it is impossible. That is to say, a woman may be least traumatized by having a Cesarean and a live baby, when a spontaneous vaginal birth is not possible. We let go of that goal to achieve the possibility of a healthy baby. Likewise, the situation in which parents may choose to allow a very ill, premature or deformed infant to die in their arms rather than being subjected to multiple surgeries, separations and ICU stays. This too, is a letting-go of the normal for the most healing choice possible, given the circumstances, within the framework of the parent's ethics. What is most healing will, of course, vary from individual to individual.

[7]We place the emphasis of our care on supporting life (preventive measures, good nutrition, emotional health, etc.) and not pathology, diagnosis, treatment of problems, and heroic solutions in an attempt to preserve life at any cost of quality.

[8]This addresses the medical model's tendency to ignore a woman's sense of well-being or danger in many aspects of health care, but particularly in regard to her pregnancy.

[9]This acknowledges that the thrust of our care centers on the mother, her health, her well-being, her nutrition, her habits and emotional balance so that, in turn, the baby benefits. This view is diametrically opposed to the medical model which often attempts to care for the fetus or baby while dismissing or even excluding the mother.

F. We value pregnancy and birth as rites of passage integral to a woman's evolution into mothering.

G. We value the potential of partners, family and community to support women in all aspects of birth and mothering.[10]

VI. The Nature of Relationship

A. We value relationships. The quality, integrity, equality and uniqueness of our interactions inform and critique our choices and decisions.

B. We value honesty in relationships.

C. We value caring for women to the best of our ability without prejudice against their age, race, religion, culture, sexual orientation, physical abilities or socioeconomic background.

D. We value the concept of personal responsibility and the right of individuals to make choices regarding what they deem best for themselves. We value the right to true informed choice, not merely informed consent, to what we think is best.

E. We value our relationship to a process larger than ourselves, recognizing that birth is something we can seek to learn from and know, but never control.

F. We value humility in our work.

G. We value the recognition of our own limits and limitations.

H. We value direct access to information readily understood by all.

I. We value sharing information and our understanding about birth experiences, skills and knowledge.

J. We value the midwifery community as a support system and an essential place of learning and sisterhood.

K. We value diversity among midwives, recognizing that it broadens our collective resources and challenges us to work for greater understanding of birth and each other.

L. We value mutual trust and respect, which grow from a realization of all of the above.

MAKING DECISIONS AND ACTING ETHICALLY

These values reflect our feelings regarding how we frame midwifery in our hearts and minds. However, due to the broad range of geographic, religious, cultural, political, educational and personal backgrounds among our membership,

---

[10]While partners, other family members and a woman's larger community can and often do provide her with vital support, in using the word *potential* we wish to acknowledge that many women find themselves pregnant and mothering in abusive and unsafe environments.

how we act based on these values will be very individual. Acting ethically is a complex merging of our values and these background influences, combined with the relationship we have to others who may be involved in the process taking place. We call upon all these resources when deciding how to respond in the moment to each situation.

We acknowledge the limitations of ethical codes that present a list of rules that must be followed, recognizing that such a code may interfere with, rather than enhance, our ability to make choices. To apply such rules, we must have moral integrity, an ability to make judgments, and adequate information; with all of these, an appeal to a code becomes superfluous. Furthermore, when we set up rigid ethical codes, we may begin to cease considering the transformations we go through as a result of our choices as well as negate our wish to foster truly diversified practice. Rules are not something we can appeal to when all else fails. This, however, is the illusion fostered by traditional codes of ethics.[11] MANA's support of the individual's moral integrity grows out of an understanding that there cannot possibly be one right answer for all situations.

We acknowledge the following basic concepts and believe that ethical judgments can be made with these thoughts in mind:

- Moral agency and integrity are born within the heart of each individual.
- Judgments are fundamentally based on awareness and understanding of ourselves and others and are primarily derived from one's own sense of moral integrity with reference to clearly articulated values. Becoming aware and increasing our understanding are ongoing processes facilitated by our efforts at personal growth on every level. The wisdom gained by this process cannot be taught or dictated, but one can learn to realize, experience and evaluate it.
- The choices we can or will actually make may be limited by the oppressive nature of the medical, legal or cultural framework in which we live. The more our values conflict with those of the dominant culture, the more risky it becomes to act truly in accord with our values.
- The pregnant woman and midwife are both individual moral agents unique to themselves, having independent value and worth.
- We support ourselves, and the women and families we serve, to follow and make known the dictates of our own consciences as our relationship begins and evolves, especially when decisions must be made that impact us or the care being provided. It is up to all of us to work out a mutually satisfactory relationship when and if that is possible.

---

[11]Sarah Lucia Hoagland, paraphrased from her book *Lesbian Ethics*.

It is useful to understand the two basic theories on which moral judgments and decision-making processes are based. These processes become particularly important when one considers that in our profession a given woman's rights may not be absolute in all cases and in certain situations the woman may not be considered autonomous or competent to make her own decisions.

One of the main theories of ethics states that one should look to the consequences of the act (that is, the outcome) and not the act itself to determine if it is appropriate care. This point of view looks for the greatest good for the greatest number. The other primary ethical theory states that one should look to the act itself (that is, type of care provided) and, if it is right, then this could override the net outcome. This is a more process-oriented, feminist perspective. As midwives, we weave these two perspectives in the process of making decisions in our practices. Since the outcome of pregnancy is ultimately unknown and is always unknowable, it is inevitable that in certain circumstances our best decisions in the moment will lead to consequences we could not foresee. In summary, acting ethically is facilitated by:

- Carefully defining our values.
- Weighing the values in consideration with those of the community of midwives, families and culture in which we find ourselves.
- Acting in accord with our values to the best of our ability as the situation demands.
- Engaging in ongoing self-examination and evaluation.

There are both individual and social implications to any decision-making process. The actual rules and oppressive aspects of a society are never exact, and therefore conflicts may arise. We must weigh which choices or obligations take precedence over others. There are inevitably times when resolution does not occur and we will be unable to make peace with any course of action or may feel conflicted about a choice already made. The community of women, both midwives and those we serve, will provide a fruitful resource for continued moral support and guidance.

BIBLIOGRAPHY

Cross, Star, MANA Ethics Chair. unpublished draft of MANA Ethics code, 1989.

Daly, Mary. *Gyn Ecology: The Metaethics of Radical Feminism*, Boston, MA: Beacon Press, 1978.

Hoagland, Sarah Lucia. *Lesbian Ethics: Toward New Value*, Palo Alto, CA: Institute of Lesbian Studies, 1988.

Johnson, Sonia. *Going out of Our Minds: The Metaphysics of Liberation*, Freedom CA: Crossing Press, 1987.

Standards and Qualifications for the Art and Practice of Midwifery

Revised at the Midwives Alliance Business Meeting October 2, 2005

The midwife practices in accord with the MANA Standards and Qualifications for the Art and Practice of Midwifery and the MANA Statement of Values and Ethics, and demonstrates the clinical skills and judgments described in the MANA Core Competencies for Midwifery Practice.

1. *Skills*—Necessary skills of a practicing midwife include the ability to:
   - Provide continuity of care to the woman and her newborn during the maternity cycle. Care may continue throughout the woman's entire life cycle. The midwife recognizes that childbearing is a woman's experience and encourages the active involvement of her self-defined family system
   - Identify, assess and provide care during the antepartal, intrapartal, postpartal, and newborn periods. She may also provide well woman and newborn care
   - Maintain proficiency in life-saving measures by regular review and practice
   - Deal with emergency situations appropriately
   - Use judgment, skill and intuition in competent assessment and response
2. *Appropriate equipment and treatment*—Midwives carry and maintain equipment to assess and provide care for the well-woman, the mother, the fetus, and the newborn; to maintain clean and/or aseptic technique; and to treat conditions including, but not limited to, hemorrhage, lacerations, and cardio-respiratory distress. This may include the use of non-pharmaceutical agents, pharmaceutical agents, and equipment for suturing and intravenous therapy.
3. *Records*—Midwives keep accurate records of care for each woman and newborn in their practice. Records shall reflect current standards in midwifery charting and shall be held confidential (except as legally required). Records shall be provided to the woman on request. The mid-

wife maintains confidentiality in all verbal and written communications regarding women in her care.

4. *Data Collection*—It is highly recommended that midwives collect data for their practice on a regular basis and that this be done prospectively, following the protocol developed by the MANA Division of Research. Data collected by the midwife shall be used to inform and improve her practice.

5. *Compliance*—Midwives will inform and assist parents regarding public health requirements of the jurisdiction in which the midwifery service is provided.

6. *Medical Consultation, Collaboration, and Referral*—All midwives recognize that there are certain conditions for which medical consultations are advisable. The midwife shall make a reasonable attempt to assure that her client has access to consultation, collaboration, and/or referral to a medical care system when indicated.

7. *Screening*—Midwives respect the woman's right to self-determination. Midwives assess and inform each woman regarding her health and well-being relevant to the appropriateness of midwifery services. It is the right and responsibility of the midwife to refuse or discontinue services in certain circumstances. Appropriate referrals are made in the interest of the mother or baby's well-being or when the required or requested care is outside the midwife's personal scope of practice as described in her practice guidelines.

8. *Informed Choice*—Each midwife will present accurate information about herself and her services, including but not limited to:
   - Her education in midwifery
   - Her experience level in midwifery
   - Her practice guidelines
   - Her financial charges for services
   - The services she does and does not provide
   - Her expectations of the pregnant woman and the woman's self-defined family system

   The midwife recognizes that the woman is the primary decision maker in all matters regarding her own health care and that of her infant.

   The midwife respects the woman's right to decline treatments or procedures and properly documents these choices. The midwife clearly states and documents when a woman's choices fall outside the midwife's practice guidelines.

9. *Continuing Education*—Midwives will update their knowledge and skills on a regular basis.

10. *Peer Review*—Midwifery practice includes an on-going process of case review with peers
11. *Practice Guidelines*—Each midwife will develop practice guidelines for her services that are in agreement with the MANA Standards and Qualifications for the Art and Practice of Midwifery, the MANA Statement of Values and Ethics, and the MANA Core Competencies for Midwifery Practice, in keeping with her level of expertise.
12. *Expanded scope of practice*—The midwife may expand her scope of practice beyond the MANA Core Competencies to incorporate new procedures that improve care for women and babies consistent with the midwifery model of care. Her practice must reflect knowledge of the new procedure, including risks, benefits, screening criteria, and identification and management of potential complications.

The following sources were utilized for reference

- Essential documents of the National Association of Certified Professional Midwives 2004
- American College of Nurse-Midwives documents and standards for the Practice of Midwifery revised March 2003
- ICM membership and joint study on maternity; FIGO, WHO, etc. revised 1972
- New Mexico regulations for the practice of lay midwifery, revised 1982
- North West Coalition of Midwives Standards for Safety and Competency in Midwifery
- Varney, Helen, *Nurse-Midwifery*, Blackwell Scientific Publishing, Boston, MA 1980

American College of Nurse-Midwives Code of Ethics with Explanatory Statements

INTRODUCTION

Certified nurse–midwives (CNMs) and certified midwives (CMs) have three ethical mandates in achieving the mission of midwifery to promote the health and well-being of women and newborns within their families and communities. The first mandate is directed toward the individual women and their families for whom the midwives provide care, the second mandate is to a broader audience for the "public good" for the benefit of all women and their families, and the third mandate is to the profession of midwifery to assure its integrity and in turn its ability to fulfill the mission of midwifery.

The *Code of Ethics of the American College of Nurse-Midwives* describes moral obligations that guide the behaviors of midwives and individuals representing the profession of midwifery, including those in the American College of Nurse Midwives (ACNM). The moral obligations reflect universal ethical principles that are traditionally associated with the health-care professions but have been written to emphasize midwifery values and standards in the various roles of professional midwifery practice: care for women and their families, education, research, public policy and the business management and financial organization of health services.

The *Code of Ethics* has three sections. The first section is devoted solely to professional relationships that midwives have with all persons. The first moral obligation sets forth the expected behavior of midwives in relation to the moral worth of all persons with whom they interact in any professional context. The second moral obligation takes into account the moral worth of midwives and how they consider themselves in all professional relationships. In view of the fact that these two moral obligations pertain to all relationships, they are foundational to all of the other nine moral obligations in the *Code of Ethics*.

The second section of the *Code of Ethics* includes the moral obligations (#3 through #9) that have relevance for midwives in their professional practice,

217

whatever that may be. These moral obligations represent ideal action to be upheld by midwives. Usually more than one moral obligation applies in a particular situation.

In the context of contemporary health care, however, ethical issues and dilemmas frequently occur. New burdens include more work to do in the allotted time, greater numbers of health-care professionals and providers with whom to interact, and the pressure of containing the financial cost of health care. The conflict of two or more moral obligations in a particular situation necessitates deliberate ethical analysis and decision making, including weighing and balancing principles and preferably involving and achieving consensus among all affected parties to determine ethically justified courses of action. In these conflicts, the moral obligations involved may be given different weights by the affected parties. Therefore, it is not possible to say that the moral obligations in this section are absolute all of the time or that one has precedence over another in all situations. It is through moral reasoning and decision making that actions may be justified as ethical to the extent that they can be in a given situation. When ethical conflicts recur, especially with similar contextual circumstances, it becomes necessary to consider what efforts might be taken to reassess the causes of the conflicts, the commitments professionals bring to the situation, and the potential for ethical compromises.

The third section focuses on what midwives do to support midwifery as a profession and the functions customarily accomplished through the ACNM to promote the public good and assure the fulfillment of the responsibilities of the profession, as described in the bylaws of the American College of Nurse-Midwives. In adhering to the moral obligations in the third section, an individual midwife shares with all other midwives a responsibility for the profession. From an ethical perspective, it is expected that all midwives will assume their fair share of the responsibility and exercise it in light of their various interests and capabilities throughout their professional careers.

In summary, through behaviors consonant with the moral obligations contained in the *Code of Ethics*, midwives support and maintain the integrity of the profession of midwifery and thus contribute to a profession worthy of being considered by society as a public good. Although the *Code of Ethics* is viewed as a document that purposefully is brief and can stand alone, it is supplemented by explanatory statements in this expanded version. Each explanatory statement is written in relation to a specific moral obligation and links ethical principles and concepts to the moral action called for by the moral obligation. The explanatory statements further clarify to whom the moral obligation is directed, specify the conditions and circumstances in which it is relevant and identify the responsibilities of midwives and the ideal moral behavior in a particular context.

This revised *Code of Ethics* has several important uses by midwives within the profession. The code serves as a guide for midwives in their professional practice in whatever roles they assume, provides a framework for peer consultation and review and orients midwifery students to the moral obligations of the profession into which they are being socialized. The code also informs others about the ethical principles that guide professional midwifery practice.

EXPLANATORY STATEMENTS

Midwives in all aspects of professional relationships will:

1. Respect basic human rights and the dignity of all persons.

Respect for basic human rights and the dignity of all persons provides the foundation for midwifery practice. Respecting human rights contributes to the maintenance and good of society and originates in the principles of respect for autonomy and justice. Respect for autonomy occurs when people are able to determine the courses of action they will take and accept accountability for the outcome of these choices. Justice occurs when people are treated fairly and equitably. Human rights are what people in a society should be able to expect in terms of how they are treated by others and how they acquire the necessities and opportunities for their well-being.

Basic human rights are universal, applying equally to men and women, and include the right to: dignity, safety or security of one's body, food and nutrition, shelter, privacy, freedom from any form of discrimination, information and education, health, and equitable access to quality health services (United Nations, 1948). Reproductive rights were added to these basic human rights in the mid-1990s and are of particular relevance to midwifery practice (Thompson, 2004). However, both basic human rights and reproductive rights have not been accorded to young girls and women globally at the same level as for young boys and men (Cook, 1994).

As midwives work primarily with women, they are in a position to support and promote the rights of women. Midwives also understand the adverse consequences that human rights violations have on the health of women and infants, such as violence, maternal death and disability, and lack of health services. Midwives have a responsibility to work to eliminate these violations on the individual level, when they affect the women for whom they provide care, and on the level of policy development and advocacy (see explanatory statements #9 and #11). These actions reflect basic tenets of midwifery practice and support the ethical principle of beneficence (by doing good while avoiding or preventing harm) as well as the principle of justice (by reducing the inequitable treatment of women).

Respecting human dignity acknowledges the humanity of all people and is the *prima facie* human right that sets the standard for all interactions among people. By respecting human dignity, the midwife upholds the ethical principle of respect for autonomy. This requires midwives to listen to, recognize and reflect on different points of view to understand any impact these differences may have on the professional relationship and the choices and outcomes of care. Respect does not imply automatic agreement with another's decision or actions, nor does it relieve midwives of the obligation to protect others and themselves when choices may cause harm (see explanatory statements #3 and #8).

This moral obligation applies to all persons with whom midwives have professional relationships, including those who receive midwifery care, members of the health-care team, administrators, policy makers and students. Trust, integrity, truth-telling, compassion, caring, and respect form the foundation for positive professional relationships.

References

Cook, R. J. (1994). *Women's health and human rights*. Geneva, Switzerland: World Health Organization.

Thompson, J. B. (2004). A human rights framework for midwifery care. *Journal of Midwifery & Women's Health, 49*(3), 175–181.

United Nations. (1948). *United Nations Charter: Universal declaration of human rights*. New York.

Midwives in all aspects of professional relationships will:

2. Respect their own self worth, dignity and professional integrity.

The call for all midwives to respect their own self worth and dignity stems from the same ethical principles, respect for autonomy, and justice, that require midwives to honor the human rights and the dignity of all people. By virtue of their humanity, midwives have worth—both per se and by virtue of their rationality, which allows them to exercise dignity in professional relationships. To respect their own self worth and dignity, midwives must understand the value and the limits of their own knowledge, beliefs and emotions in professional interactions. In decision making, this sense of self worth ensures that they safeguard their own dignity, just as they strive to safeguard the dignity of others.

Although "self" is primarily used in this moral obligation to emphasize that midwives have equal status with other human beings, the concept of self-worth reflects how midwives respect their own dignity. The self-worth of midwives is in part based on their ability to respect their own values and competences in interaction with others and seek alternative solutions to prevent compromise of important professional principles, values and goals. In negotiating the tension between "self" and "other," midwives have to balance their need for professional autonomy and recognition of their knowledge and skills with the competing needs for autonomy of the "other," be that a client, administrator or colleague who maintains a different perspective. Such cases require a delicate balancing act, often aided by some reframing of both positions.

Midwives respect their professional integrity by consistently adhering to professional standards. When professional integrity is threatened—by any situation that erodes midwives' ability to wholly support the values of the profession—they should act responsibly to achieve ethically justifiable solutions. Contemporary practice challenges midwives to reconcile longstanding ideals of the profession with the changing goals and structures of the institutions in which they practice. Perseverance may be required to affect long-term solutions. The midwifery profession, like other health-care professions, reassesses its commitments through organizational mechanisms for confirming or altering professional commitments to meet new challenges. Thus, midwives have the responsibility to continuously assess the consistency of their practice with the expectations of the profession and to participate in decision-making regarding changes. Exercising such professional integrity maximizes the profession's fit into the contemporary health-care system even as it increases the resonance between the midwives' practice and the standards of their profession. Exercising professional integrity is the best way to demonstrate respect for women who place their trust in the profession of midwifery.

The professional integrity of midwives is not to be confused with personal integrity, which is based on an individual set of values. In the course of providing health care, midwives' personal values may conflict with certain decisions of women and their families. Respecting diversity in values preserves the dignity of all parties. Midwives have the responsibility to practice with self-awareness—to understand their values and to examine their actions for any potential bias. The principle of respect for diversity should not, however, require midwives to diminish their personal or professional integrity by participating in care that sharply conflicts with their own personal values. Such situations are often best resolved through consultation with colleagues, transferring care to another health-care provider or consultation with an organizational or institutional ethics board.

References

Beauchamp, T. L., & Childress, J. F. (1994). *Principles of biomedical ethics* (4th ed.). New York: Oxford University Press.

Croker, J. (2002). The costs of seeking self-esteem. *Journal of Social Issues, 58*(3), 597–615.

Halfon, M. S. (1989). *Integrity: A philosophical inquiry.* Philadelphia: Temple University Press.

Harter, S., Walters, P., & Whitesell, N. (1998). Relational self-worth: Differences in perceived worth as a person across interpersonal contexts. *Child Development, 69*(3), 757–777.

Midwives in all aspects of their professional practice will:

3. Develop a partnership with the woman in which each shares relevant information that leads to informed decision-making, consent to an evolving plan of care, and acceptance of responsibility for the outcome of their choices.

Respect for autonomy is basic to midwifery care and is developed within a partnership that fosters open communication between a midwife and a woman. Midwives strive to include women in the process of their care and create a partnership that enables each person to maintain respect for the other and for the other's autonomy in the decision-making process. Within this partnership, a woman has the responsibility to share information about herself and her health and the right to determine the extent of her participation in the decision-making process. Midwives have the responsibility to help the woman and her family overcome any sense of dependence on the midwife and to achieve as much control within the process as is desired and possible.

Midwives also strive to make clear the expectation of mutual responsibility in the partnership for choosing a course of action and the resulting outcome, including transfer of care. They also are responsible for disclosing any conflict or bias they may have toward the information provided, options given, and the extent to which they must limit or refuse participation in a particular course of action. The partnership between a woman and a midwife may be ended by either party. Some limits to this partnership include the development of an intimate relationship (as defined by state laws and regulations) and criminal activity.

Midwives and women share relevant information. The quality of care provided by midwives depends in part on this mutual sharing of information. This information should be relevant, accurate, truthful and reflect the uniqueness of the woman and her family. Midwives are responsible for describing the standard of clinical care that is applicable to the situation, the credentials and limitations of the practitioner providing the care, and providing for the seamless continuation of care if the need exceeds their qualifications.

Midwives also obtain consent to an evolving plan of care. This includes but is not limited to written consent for general treatment and any specific invasive procedure. Consent given through participatory behavior may be acceptable for non-invasive forms of treatment. The following are three key concepts necessary in obtaining consent for a mutually agreeable plan of care: 1) disclosure of information including risks, benefits and care options; 2) clarification that the woman understands that information; and 3) assurance of the voluntary nature of the consent. Midwives have the responsibility to explore the woman's understanding of and her ability to articulate the information provided, as well as to consider cultural and social influences in the interpretation of information shared. It is also their responsibility to ensure to the degree possible that a woman's consent is given freely and is not constrained by the undue influence of family members, the midwife or other care-providers, or other aspects of the environment. Factors that can threaten the voluntary nature of consent are problems with funding for care, lack of privacy when the information is disclosed, expectations related to research alternatives (see explanatory statement #8), limitations on access to other practitioners, and involvement in an abusive relationship. Giving informed and voluntary consent leads a higher degree of ownership of decisions for the woman. Ownership of health-care decisions helps women live with and accept the personal realities of their choices. Therefore, midwives work diligently to ensure that women own their decisions to the maximum degree possible.

Midwives and women share responsibility for the outcome of their choices. The ethical principles of beneficence (to do good) and nonmaleficence (to do no harm) are partners with respect for autonomy. The goal of a professional relationship between a midwife and a woman is to arrive at a plan of care that optimizes the woman's health through informed decision making, is consistent with professional standards of practice, and is acceptable to both. All these conditions are necessary in order for each to accept responsibility for the outcome of clinical decisions. Midwives have the professional responsibility to do no harm; and if a woman's choice endangers herself or others, midwives are obligated to preserve their professional integrity as well as to promote the welfare of the family. This responsibility requires midwives to explain this limit to women at the outset of the partnership and may at times necessitate clinical management that is not a woman's first choice.

References

Beauchamp, T. L., & Childress, J. F. (2001). *Principles of biomedical ethics* (5th ed.). New York: Oxford University Press.

Mackenzie, C., & Stoljar, N. (Eds.). *Relational autonomy: Feminist perspectives on autonomy, agency, and the social self*. New York: Oxford University Press.

Wolf, S. M. (Ed.). (1996). *Feminism & bioethics*. New York: Oxford University Press.

Midwives in all aspects of their own professional practice will:

4. Act without discrimination based on factors such as age, gender, race, ethnicity, religion, lifestyle, sexual orientation, socioeconomic status, disability, or nature of the health problem.

Midwives strive for equality and justice in all aspects of their clinical and professional activity and must respect the rights of all people. They have the responsibility to act without discrimination by avoiding differential and negative treatment of individuals on the basis of their age, gender, race, ethnicity, religion, lifestyle, sexual orientation, socioeconomic status, disability, group membership, or the nature of their health problem. Midwives strive to provide appropriate care regardless of the restrictions or difficulties encountered. Providing appropriate care requires midwives to become familiar with cultural expectations that may affect both the quality and expected outcome of heath care. This includes their own opinions and behaviors and those of others that may inhibit women from exercising autonomy in making health-care choices.

Discrimination within federal, state, and institutional systems has a major influence on the ability of midwives to provide care. Discrimination can vary from complicated patient forms to institutional barriers, including a lack of availability of culturally acceptable food services or a lack of access to operating room and specialized services. Organizational hazards can influence the quality of women's health care by causing difficulties in accessing a social benefit and bias in the structure of decision-making processes within the institution or practice setting. Midwives become the woman's advocate when institutional decisions about allocation of resources must be made.

Respect for justice is a crucial ethical principle that can apply at many levels in the health-care system. The right to health care is a claim that individuals justly make. Justice requires that midwives promote health and the provision of quality heath care that provides equal opportunity in access and quality for all people. This may mean advocating for change in the political structure (see explanatory statement #9). Acting without discrimination means that midwives perform all aspects of their professional practice without treating women differently because of bias about any special characteristic.

Midwives must respect the rights of all people regardless of the nature of the health problem. Discrimination is inferred to underlie the observed health disparities among different groups' risks of infant and maternal mortality and morbidity. Those segments of the population most vulnerable in the United States are: high-risk mothers and infants; people with chronic illness, disabilities, AIDS, or mental illness; people with alcohol or substance dependence; people living with domestic violence; homeless women; women of color; and immigrants, refugees and incarcerated women. In particular, midwives must be cognizant of their own bias and take appropriate action to assess the equality of health care they provide.

References

Callahan, D. (2002). Ends and means: The goals of health care. In M. Danus, C. Clancy, & L. R. Churchill (Eds.), *Ethical dimensions of health policy* (pp. 3–47). New York: Oxford University Press.

Krieger N. (2002). Discrimination and health. In L. F. Berkman & I. Kawachi (Eds.), *Social epidemiology* (pp. 36–75). New York: Oxford University Press.

Smedley, B. D., Stith, A. Y., & Nelson, A. R. (Eds.). (2000). *Unequal treatment: Confronting racial and ethnic disparities in health care*. Washington, DC: The National Academies. Available from: http://www.iom.edu/repot.asp?id+4475.

Midwives in all aspects of their professional practice will:

5. Provide an environment where privacy is protected and in which all pertinent information is shared without bias, coercion, or deception.

The partnership between the woman and the midwife occurs within an environment that impacts the quality of the relationship, whether that environment is influenced by governmental sources, practice setting or reimbursement agencies. The obligation of the profession to set and monitor its own ethical standards requires midwives to be aware of and change where possible any external factors that adversely affect the privacy or veracity of information provided.

Protecting the privacy and veracity of the woman's medical record is provided for under the Health Insurance Portability and Accountability Act, known as HIPAA. This law serves to protect the medical information of patients as it is transferred between agencies. Besides being responsible for ensuring that the legal aspects of this act are known and observed, midwives correct other conditions in the environment that may breach the privacy of the medical record. These conditions include but are not limited to: open and visible computer screens, identifiable names in public places, e-mails, faxes and unfiled or unsecured medical records.

Protecting the personal privacy of the woman within the setting where care is rendered can often be challenging, whether this occurs in the hospital, office or home. Midwives are expected to respect the woman's choice of people who may invade that privacy, including hospital personnel, and her choice of location for disclosing sensitive information. In situations where inadequate physical protective barriers affect the woman's privacy, midwives strive to improve those conditions.

Sharing of pertinent information with bias, coercion or deception can threaten a woman's autonomy. The midwife's awareness of the environment in which care is rendered can help her to avoid bias, coercion and deception that may come from an institution's philosophical rules, funding sources and advertising. Since the information that a midwife provides to women may be influenced by such factors, she works to be aware of them, particularly where medications and treatment options are involved, and states clearly to the woman where the bias occurs, including any personal bias.

Sharing of pertinent information through a language barrier, whether a translator is used or not, deserves particular attention. If a third party is involved in the translation, midwives need to assess the veracity of translation and the understanding of the woman. Particular attention needs to be paid when the translator is a child, as the woman may be reluctant or find it impossible to discuss information of a sexual or reproductive nature in a child's presence.

Midwives in all aspects of their professional practice will:
6. Maintain confidentiality except where disclosure is mandated by law.

In health care, much attention has been given to confidentiality between patients and providers. Maintaining confidentiality extends beyond women to their families and others with whom midwives interact professionally and socially. This obligation is based on respect for autonomy (because individuals make decisions about how information about them will be used) and is the foundation of fidelity and trust in all patient-provider relationships.

Maintaining confidentiality means that information exchanged between the woman and midwife is given with either explicit or implicit understanding that it will not be disclosed to others unless specific permission is given by the woman. Information may be received verbally from the woman, from her physical examination and laboratory tests, or with the woman's consent, through a third source. A violation of confidentiality occurs when any information is disclosed without consent, regardless of the benefit or harm. It is the real or perceived harm caused by disclosure that midwives wish to prevent.

Disclosure of confidential information may be necessary when that information has the potential to result in harm to the woman or others. Whenever possible, these circumstances should be discussed with the woman prior to the exchange of information. Such departures are not taken lightly and have to be considered in the context of the principle of nonmaleficence (which seeks to avoid inflicting harm) and the principle of beneficence (since preventing harm is a form of doing good). Each state has specific requirements for reporting information mandated by law, and midwives need to be familiar with these statutes. Exceptions to the maintenance of confidentiality include but are not limited to suicidal threats or attempts, reportable infectious diseases, gunshot wounds and child abuse.

Justification for disclosure of information that is not covered by legal statute commonly emerges when women or third parties face serious danger. Under these circumstances the obligation to protect from harm may override the woman's right to autonomy. When faced with a conflict between a woman's right to autonomy and the responsibility to avoid harm, midwives should consider consulting with colleagues directly involved in that care and seek others with expertise directly related to the conflict.

The midwife has a responsibility to remain current with ethical debates concerning disclosure of sensitive information to a third party, which may not be explicitly covered by legal statute and for which there is a lack of sufficient evidence or consensus for breaching confidentiality. Legal and moral rules for confidentiality are still evolving in response to HIV disease and genetic testing, for example. Midwives are expected to encourage the woman to share information with those at risk for infection or a genetic condition; but as long as the third person's life is not in imminent danger, there is insufficient evidence to support breaching confidentiality.

Midwives in all aspects of their professional practice will:
7. Maintain the necessary knowledge, skills and behaviors needed for competence.

Competence, an important ethical concept, requires the adaptation and integration of knowledge and skills into the behaviors needed in a particular context. The specific nature of a midwife's work determines what constitutes competence and therefore determines the knowledge, skills, and behaviors to be maintained by a midwife. The behaviors indicative of competence differ among midwives because of the diversity of professional work settings. Maintaining competence in all aspects of professional practice includes clinical practice, teaching, administration, research, and consultation, whether these are practiced singly or in combination.

Competence is dynamic, not static. Rapid changes in the knowledge and skills of midwifery and related disciplines, changes in society, and changes in available health-care resources all force the definition of competence to evolve. By being competent, midwives assure their ability to contribute to the good of others and to prevent harm while also preserving their own integrity and that of the midwifery profession.

Expectations for the behaviors that compose competence are articulated through standards established by the ACNM and other standard-setting bodies. The necessary knowledge, skills and behaviors for midwives' actual practice are specific to current professional standards and the context in which the midwives practice

All midwives graduate with beginning competence in midwifery and the expectation that they will engage in self-assessment and lifelong learning to maintain currency in the knowledge and skills necessary for their particular work. Demonstrating behaviors that represent competence promotes midwives' professional honesty as well as their trustworthiness to women and their families, their colleagues and the profession.

Midwives in all aspects of their professional practice will:
8. Protect women, their families and colleagues from harmful, unethical and incompetent practices by taking appropriate action that may include reporting as mandated by law.

Effective practice requires that midwives assume responsibility not only for the competence of their own behavior but for competence in the broader context of their practice settings. The ethical principles of nonmaleficence and of beneficence underlie this moral obligation, as they do many of the obligations described in this document, but here beneficence refers specifically to the prevention of or protection from harm, rather than the more general meaning of doing or promoting good (Beauchamp & Childress, 2001, p.115). Except in rare instances when causing some harm is necessary to prevent a more severe harm, midwives should avoid causing harm to themselves or others. Harm, in this context, means adverse physical, emotional, psychological, social or economic effects of practices or behaviors. Incompetent or unethical actions may result in harm and may occur in any area of midwives' professional practice: clinical practice, administration, business practice, education and research. Midwives assume this responsibility to protect not only the women and families for whom they provide care, but also those for whom their colleagues provide care. Midwives, in turn, assume responsibility to protect themselves and their colleagues from practices or behaviors that may cause harm. The action taken by the midwife depends on the circumstances of the harmful or potentially harmful practice. When an unethical and incompetent practice is likely to cause harm, midwives should try to prevent it from occurring by working through existing systems to support established and current clinical standards. If, however, a harmful practice is in process, midwives must take action to interrupt, terminate or mitigate the practice. This may require working within different administrative, institutional or legal systems.

Midwives are responsible to protect women, their families and colleagues from harmful, unethical and incompetent behavior in clinical practice settings. The inability to adhere to standards of clinical practice may result from a lack of knowledge and skill; mental, physical and emotional impairment affecting judgment and application of skills; drug or alcohol abuse; or a deliberate (knowing and willing) decision to violate standards. Impaired midwives must seek assistance and either take action to regain the ability to practice safely or withdraw from practice. Colleagues of midwives unable to provide care seek to provide a seamless transfer of care for the women and families affected. Midwives also need to be aware of policies and laws that apply to their practice environment and identify and report any unsafe conditions. Midwives correct unsafe conditions for which they have responsibility and report those for which they do not have immediate responsibility.

Midwives also guard against harmful, unethical, and incompetent behavior in business practices. Business practices deal not only with the operation of a clinical practice but also with other areas of professional practice and organization. Therefore, all midwives will have some responsibility related to business practices, but the responsibility is greater for midwives who have oversight for the financial aspects of a service, facility or funded grants or contracts. It is the responsibility of the midwife to know the statutes, regulations and business standards that govern practice and avoid breach of contract. Midwives strive to present accurate information about the health-care services they provide. Midwives also should not accept financial incentives from payers for the provision of services or monetary or other types of gifts from outside companies.

Midwives also avoid harmful, unethical, and incompetent practices in education. Midwifery faculty have the responsibility to educate midwives to be competent to begin practice in midwifery. Midwives who engage in teaching students have responsibilities to the students as well as to the women for whom they care. Midwives and their students must provide safe care to fully informed clients, in a manner that respects the boundaries of the relationship between student and faculty. In addition, midwives and their students should promote intellectual honesty in their teaching and learning.

Finally, midwives protect women, their families and colleagues from harmful, unethical, and incompetent practices in research. Midwives assume various obligations pertaining to research. They may be caring for women or teaching students who are potential subjects for research, conducting their own research, or serving as consultants, peer reviewers and members of research review boards. Midwives who conduct research or serve as a peer reviewer of research proposals and reports are responsible for assuring that the research is scientifically and ethically sound and may benefit the participants and population from which the research subjects are drawn. Midwives participating in research or providing access to clients are responsible for insuring that research subjects are fully informed about the research and their rights as research subjects. Records of subjects must be maintained so that they can be contacted if untoward effects are later discovered, and any such effects must be reported. Midwives who are part of a research team are responsible for the accuracy and completeness of the data. Midwives who are principal investigators or part of the research team involved in the data analysis are responsible for the integrity of the analysis and reported results. Furthermore, midwives are obligated not to engage in research solely for financial gain or personal reward. In sum, the principles of honesty, veracity, trust, fidelity, and justice that span many of the other moral obligations described in this document also support actions that prevent harm.

Reference

Beauchamp, T. L., & Childress, J. F. (2001). *Principles of biomedical ethics* (5th ed.). New York: Oxford University Press.

Midwives as members of a profession will:
9. Promote, advocate for, and strive to protect the rights, health, and well-being of women, families and communities.

The midwifery profession has unique expertise and experience in providing care for women, especially during the childbearing years. In recognition of that expertise, midwives have a responsibility to take actions to promote (by working actively), to advocate for (by speaking and writing in support of), and to strive to protect (by defending) the rights, health and well-being of the women, families and communities they serve. This responsibility extends beyond women to their families and communities because women's health and well-being are so strongly tied to the people and conditions around them.

This moral obligation requires that midwives go beyond individual actions to represent midwifery within broader political and societal structures at local, regional, national and international levels. Through their actions, midwives promote and advocate for changes in social structures, programs, regulations and laws that would enhance the rights, health and well-being of women, families and communities, while also protecting the safeguards that already exist.

The rights identified in this moral obligation are the same human rights defined in the first moral obligation. As with the previous obligations this document describes, the responsibilities of this moral obligation go beyond basic human rights to include health and well-being which are fundamental needs.

Midwives also have an obligation to support the ACNM to fulfill the profession's responsibilities in this matter. Midwives can support the ACNM across a continuum of activities, from providing input into policy and advocacy decisions to responding to requests for comments, participating in forums for discussion, or taking a leadership role within the organization. In such roles, midwives "speak for" midwifery and not as individuals.

The actions and positions that midwives and the professional organization take to fulfill this moral obligation should be driven by the public good (the rights, health and well-being of women, families and communities), not the goal of promoting, advocating for or protecting the profession of midwifery alone. Members take on the additional responsibility to ensure that the actions and positions of the ACNM continue to reflect the intent of this obligation. As social, cultural, economic and political conditions change, midwives and their professional organization will need to explore, question, reconfirm and revise position statements.

Reference

Bayles, M. D. (1989). *Professional ethics* (2nd ed.). Belmont, CA: Wadsworth, 166–184.

Midwives as members of a profession will:

10. Promote just distribution of resources and equity in access to quality health services.

Because of their knowledge of the health-care needs of women and their families, promoting the allocation of resources justly and equitably among population groups is a responsibility of midwives. Midwives need to collaborate with others to create the political will and advocacy for just and equitable budget allocations.

While this moral obligation relates to explanatory statements nine and eleven, it commands separate attention because of its unique emphasis on justness and equity in the allocation of resources to population groups, often referred to as macroallocation. This encompasses the development of policies that establish how resources for health care will be distributed. More just and equitable distribution of basic human resources enhances the ability of midwives and others to provide a higher quality of health services.

The concept of quality health care services has broad interest and support. It is predicated on the beliefs that access to health care is a human right, that the health-care needs of individuals should be met, and that the dignity and autonomy of individuals should be honored in receiving and providing care. In the United States, the Institute of Medicine has identified six dimensions of health-care services that contribute to their quality: safety, effectiveness, patient centeredness, timeliness, efficiency and equity (Institute of Medicine, 2001). All these dimensions are affected by the characteristics and availability of resources. Policies and funding determine how health-care personnel, facilities for health care, and access to affordable health care are defined.

When quality health-care services cannot be adequately supported because of scarce resources, justness and equity should guide policy deliberations over macroallocation. Justness, in terms of fairness, is achieved when health-care resources are made available similarly to individuals across public and/or private health-care systems. Equity is achieved not when all individuals with particular health-related characteristics are included in health services but when all individuals with similar characteristics are provided for similarly. Withholding health care because of personal attributes is considered unfair customarily. Examples of equity in women's health care include equal access to comprehensive maternity care for all women of reproductive age and evidence-based diagnostic and treatment services for all women with breast cancer. However, scarce resources might not be allocated for treatment of a condition with an uncertain or low probability of cure.

Attention to the macroallocation of health-care resources is an ongoing process that, in the context of economic constraints, aims to maximize the availability of resources in proportion to the needs of the populations to be served.

The policy decisions made in relation to macroallocation directly influence the resources available to individual patients for whom midwives and others provide direct care. Therefore, all health-care providers have a stake in the process of the just and equitable distribution of health-care resources.

Reference

Committee on Quality of Health Care in America, Institute of Medicine. (2001). *Crossing the quality divide: A new health system for the 21st century*. Washington, DC: National Academy Press, 5–6.

Midwives as members of a profession will:
11. Promote and support the education of midwifery students and peers, standards of practice, research and policies that enhance the health of women, families and communities.

Health in this moral obligation is defined broadly as a state of complete physical, mental and social well-being, not merely the absence of disease or infirmity. The profession of midwifery plays an important role in enhancing the health of women, families and communities in four interrelated areas: education of midwifery students and peers, setting of standards of practice, conducting and evaluating research, and shaping public, professional and institutional policy. Standards of practice should be driven by research and form the backbone of education; policies should be consistent with the research findings that shape standards of practice; and education should support standards of care and include skills to understand and to conduct research. The responsibility of this obligation extends beyond women to their families and communities because the health of women is so strongly tied to the people and social, cultural and economic conditions around them.

Some midwives support the education of midwifery students by serving as faculty and clinical preceptors for midwifery educational programs. All midwives have the responsibility to practice according to recognized standards of care and participate in the process of updating them when necessary. Also, all midwives need to support their professional organization and its designated certifying and accrediting bodies as these organizations fulfill their functions.

Some midwives, by virtue of their expertise and positions, contribute to the scientific knowledge base through research or participate in the development of policies that enhance the health of women, families and communities. Midwives fulfill this obligation by becoming researchers, by participating as subjects in research, by providing opportunities for the women and families they serve to participate in research, and by serving on peer review and policy-making panels and boards. When serving on policy-making panels and boards, midwives need to remember that they are addressing policy issues on behalf of midwifery or the professional organization. In short, they are "speaking for" midwifery and not as individuals.

ACNM supports research and policy development by providing direct funding, by soliciting funds to support related activities that the organization cannot support alone, and by supporting (financially and philosophically) the participation of midwives on research peer review panels, on governmental policy-making boards, and other policy-making and research related organizations. While all midwives may not directly be involved in research and policy-making, all have the responsibility to support their professional organization' s activities related to this obligation. In addition, all midwives are responsible for bringing to the attention of the profession's researchers and policy-makers issues of relevance to midwifery that may need research and policy reform.

While all of these responsibilities related to education, standards, research and policy involve midwifery as a profession, enhancement of the profession is not the primary purpose. Midwives need to engage in activities with candor and independence so that the result of their work is driven by the public good (the rights, health and well-being of women, families and communities). Therefore, midwives as members of their professional organization, ACNM, and as members of other professional organizations take on the additional responsibility to ensure that the actions and positions of their professional organizations reflect the intent of this obligation.

Reference

Bayles, M. D. (1989). *Professional ethics* (2nd ed.). Belmont, CA: Wadsworth, 166–184.

The development of this document was supported, in part, by the A.C.N.M. Foundation, Inc.
© American College of Nurse-Midwives
Silver Spring, MD 20910
Source: Ad hoc Committee to Revise the Code of Ethics
Approved: Board of Directors, 2005
Reviewed and Endorsed by the ACNM Ethics Committee, October 2008

ACKNOWLEDGMENTS

ACNM Ethics Committee

Elizabeth S. Sharp, CNM, MSN, DrPH, FACNM, FAAN, *Chairperson 2007–2010*
Robyn Brancoto, SNM, *Non-voting Member*
Katy Dawley, CNM, PhD, *Member*
Debra Hein, CNM, MSN, *Member*
Mary K. Collins, CNM, MN, *Member*

Nancy Jo Reedy, CNM, MPH, FACNM, *Member*
Kathleen E. Powderly, CNM, MSN, PhD, *Member*
Joyce E. Thompson, CNM, DrPH, FACNM, FAAN, *Member*
Leslie Ludka, CNM, *Liaison from ACNM National Office Staff 2007–2010*

Editorial Assistance
Amy Benson Brown, PhD

ICM International Code of Ethics for Midwives

'(A code of ethics) is not a dry dusty piece of paper; it is a living breathing embodiment of the spirit of midwifery and we are the ones that make it not only live, but sing and dance with the joy of life itself'

Bronwin Pelvin
New Zealand Midwife
Journal of NZCOM, 1992

PREAMBLE

The aim of the International Confederation of Midwives (ICM) is to improve the standard of care provided to women, babies and families throughout the world through the development, education, and appropriate utilization of the professional midwife. In keeping with its aim of women's health and focus on the midwife, the ICM sets forth the following code to guide the education, practice and research of the midwife. This code acknowledges women as persons with human rights, seeks justice for all people and equity in access to health care, and is based on mutual relationships of respect, trust, and the dignity of all members of society.

INTRODUCTION

In an effort to increase understanding and, hence, use of the International Code of Ethics for Midwives (1999), the ICM Board of Management commissioned the publication of this document. The document contains:

- the Code of Ethics,
- the glossary of terms used in the Code,

- the ethical analysis of the Code,
- a brief history of the development of the Code, and
- suggestions on how the midwife can use this Code in practice, education or research.

THE CODE

I. Midwifery Relationships
    A. Midwives respect a woman's informed right of choice and promote the woman's acceptance of responsibility for the outcomes of her choices.
    B. Midwives work with women, supporting their right to participate actively in decisions about their care, and empowering women to speak for themselves on issues affecting the health of women and their families in their culture/society.
    C. Midwives, together with women, work with policy and funding agencies to define women's needs for health services and to ensure that resources are fairly allocated considering priorities and availability.
    D. Midwives support and sustain each other in their professional roles, and actively nurture their own and others' sense of self-worth.
    E. Midwives work with other health professionals, consulting and referring as necessary when the woman's need for care exceeds the competencies of the midwife.
    F. Midwives recognise the human interdependence within their field of practice and actively seek to resolve inherent conflicts.
    G. The midwife has responsibilities to her or himself as a person of moral worth, including duties of moral self-respect and the preservation of integrity.
II. Practice of Midwifery
    A. Midwives provide care for women and childbearing families with respect for cultural diversity while also working to eliminate harmful practices within those same cultures.
    B. Midwives encourage realistic expectations of childbirth by women within their own society, with the minimum expectation that no women should be harmed by conception or childbearing.
    C. Midwives use their professional knowledge to ensure safe birthing practices in all environments and cultures.
    D. Midwives respond to the psychological, physical, emotional and spiritual needs of women seeking health care, whatever their circumstances.
    E. Midwives act as effective role models in health promotion for women throughout their life cycle, for families and for other health professionals.

    F. Midwives actively seek personal, intellectual and professional growth throughout their midwifery career, integrating this growth into their practice.

III. The Professional Responsibilities of Midwives

    A. Midwives hold in confidence client information in order to protect the right to privacy, and use judgement in sharing this information.

    B. Midwives are responsible for their decisions and actions, and are accountable for the related outcomes in their care of women.

    C. Midwives may refuse to participate in activities for which they hold deep moral opposition; however, the emphasis on individual conscience should not deprive women of essential health services.

    D. Midwives understand the adverse consequences that ethical and human rights violations have on the health of women and infants, and will work to eliminate these violations.

    E. Midwives participate in the development and implementation of health policies that promote the health of all women and childbearing families.

IV. Advancement of Midwifery Knowledge and Practice

    A. Midwives ensure that the advancement of midwifery knowledge is based on activities that protect the rights of women as persons.

    B. Midwives develop and share midwifery knowledge through a variety of processes, such as peer review and research.

    C. Midwives participate in the formal education of midwifery students and midwives.

Acknowledgements:
Dr. Joyce E. Thompson, CNM, DrPH
Dr. Henry O. Thompson, M.Div, PhD
Sister Anne Thompson, MTD, MS
Members of the International Confederation of Midwives Executive Committee 1990/1993 and the Delegates from member associations attending the International Council meeting in May 1993 and May 1999.

Adopted May 1993
Revised May 1999

GLOSSARY OF TERMS USED IN THE ICM INTERNATIONAL CODE OF ETHICS FOR MIDWIVES

It is the goal of the ICM that this Code of Ethics be used and tested for its relevance to the practice of midwifery and for midwives. One element of understanding relates to the use of language across cultures and societies. Therefore, the following terms are defined as used in the Code:

- **equity in access to health care** (preamble): this implies fairness in the allocation of limited resources according to need; for example, vulnerable populations/groups could receive more attention to their health needs and access to services than those who can purchase such services anywhere.

- **(health consequences of) ethical and human rights violations** (III.D.): when women are used by others, lack the freedom to make their own decisions, lack access to safe homes or education, their health will diminish.

- **human interdependence** (I.F.): since midwives work in relationship with women and others and may not always agree about what is right or should be done in a given situation, it is important that midwives seek to understand the reasons for the disagreements with clients or colleagues. Midwives do not stop with understanding or respect, however. They also work to resolve those conflicts that need to be resolved in order for ethical care to continue.

- **individual conscience** (III.C.): defined as thoughtful reflection on, analysis, and ownership of deeply held moral positions; in this context, the midwife can refuse to provide care only if someone else is available to provide the needed care.

- **informed** right of choice (I.A.): "informed" implies that complete information is given to and understood by the woman regarding the risks, benefits and probable outcomes of each choice available to her.

- **person of moral worth** (I.G.): every human being is worthy of respect and basic rights that should not be violated. The midwife should demand respect for her/himself while also respecting others.

- **professional** (Preamble): this term is used to recognise the concept that to be ethical is to be professional, to be unethical is to be unprofessional; a role recognised within one's society and accorded respect for specialised knowledge

- **professional** knowledge (II.C.): this implies midwifery knowledge gained from both formal and informal educational opportunities that lead to competence in practice.

- **professional** responsibilities (III.B.): this refers to the broad ethical duties/ obligations of the midwife that are not practice, education or research specific.

- **related** outcomes (III.C.): midwives are responsible for the results of their own decisions and actions; they cannot be held responsible for outcomes over which they have no control (e.g., genetics). There may be situations in which the midwife is ordered by someone in power to practice in an unethical manner.

We appreciate the difficulty of this situation, but the action remains unethical if the midwife chooses to follow such an order. The midwife must be aware of the risks in choosing not to follow such an order, however.

- **rights of women as persons** (Preamble and IV.A.): human rights related to any research activity including maintaining privacy, respect, telling the truth, doing good and not harming autonomy and informed consent.

- **throughout the life cycle** (II.E.); midwifery care is more than care related to childbearing; midwives care for women of all ages, many of whom never conceive or bear children; use of this phrase is an attempt to cover both reproductive and gynaecological health care for women.

- **women as persons** (Preamble); women are to be treated with respect for their being humans (not as objects or things to be used and controlled). Principles of truth-telling, privacy, autonomy and informed consent, doing good and not harming should direct any interaction between women and midwives.

ETHICAL ANALYSIS OF THE CODE OF ETHICS

Introduction

Ethics codes are often a mix of universal ethical principles and strongly held values specific to the "professional group". Below is a brief analysis of the major ethical principles and concepts that form the basis for each of the statements of the *ICM International Code of Ethics for Midwives (1999)*.

I.   Midwifery Relationships
    A. Autonomy and accountability of women; right to make choices
    B. Autonomy and "human equalities" of women; empowered to speak for herself
    C. Justice/fairness in the allocation of resources
    D. Respect for human dignity; viewing herself as a worthy individual
    E. Competence, interdependence of health professionals, safety
    F. Respect for one another
    G. Moral self-respect, dignity

II. Practice of Midwifery
    A. Respect for others, do good, do not harm
    B. Client accountability for decisions, do not harm, safety
    C. Safety; cultural relevance
    D. Respect for human dignity, treat women as whole persons

  E. Health promotion: attain/maintain autonomy, good/no harm, allocation of
   resources

  F. Competence in practice

III. Professional Responsibilities of Midwives

  A. Confidentiality; privacy

  B. Midwife accountability

  C. Midwife conscience clause: autonomy and respect of human qualities of
   the midwife

  D. Prevent human rights violations

  E. Health policy development: justice, do good

IV. Advancement of Midwifery Knowledge and Practice

  A. Protect rights of women as persons

  B. Midwife accountability, safety, competence

  C. Professional responsibility: enhance competence of all professionals to
   do good, do not harm

THE PROCESS OF DEVELOPMENT OF THE ICM CODE

The charge to develop a code of ethics that defined the moral context of
midwifery in meeting the needs of women came from the ICM Board of Management during the mid-1980s. A brief history of the process of development of
the *ICM International Code of Ethics for Midwives* may help the reader to understand more fully how specific principles and concepts were included and
why others were not. The Code was drafted in a series of workshops, beginning
in May 1986 in Vancouver, Canada and continuing in 1987 in The Hague, The
Netherlands and in 1991 in Madrid, Spain.

The final draft, the consensus document from the Executive Committee
meeting held in Madrid, was presented to the ICM Council in Vancouver, Canada,
and adopted on 6 May 1993.

Code development began with a review of systems of ethics, an understanding of how individuals develop morally, and a brief review of the history of
code development in medicine and nursing. This was followed by an analysis of
the values inherent in the ICM Constitution's statements on the aim and objectives of the Confederation, the International Definition of a Midwife
(ICM/WHO/FIGO), accepted ICM position statements as of 1992 and existing
codes of ethics from member associations.

In order to provide a world-wide (global) focus to the ICM Code, the development group aimed at statements that were often broader in their meaning
than individual association codes so that cultural/societal or ethnic variations
could be respected. Seven midwifery associations' codes of ethics received at

ICM headquarters during 1991 were analysed, revealing the following ethical concerns:

> Safety, competence, accountability, confidentiality, appropriate consultation and re-
> ferral, respect for human dignity, client involvement in decisions, participation in
> knowledge development in midwifery and the design of maternal-child health poli-
> cies, respectful interaction with other team members, health promotion, justice/
> fairness, non-discrimination, and the education of future midwives.

At all times, the concern for understandability (in the three languages of the Confederation), culturally sensitive wording, and the global nature of the ICM Code were kept in mind. Two other important features were agreed: first, that whenever possible, the ICM Code would promote a global (universal) level of morality; that is, the statements would be made reflecting universal ethical principles, with reasonable consideration for personal and/or legal authority. In keeping with this first agreement, the second was to consciously exclude reference to the law or legal entities within the Code. While ethics and law are related, the law varies from country to country. Normally, ethics or ethical systems respect the law, but at times ethics may go beyond the law.

As noted during the introduction to this document, the *ICM International Code of Ethics for Midwives* is intended to be a "living" document, and the ICM welcomes comments and suggestions for enhancing the understanding and usefulness of this document over the years.

The ICM International Code of Ethics for Midwives was revised and reconfirmed at the meeting of the International Council in May 1999, in Manila, The Philippines.

SOME QUESTIONS ABOUT A CODE OF ETHICS

1) What is a Code of Ethics?

A code of ethics is a public declaration of the beliefs and values of a profession and the members of that profession. This code makes public the goals, values and morals of those who call themselves "midwives"—a statement to the public about what the profession of midwifery defines as moral behaviour for its practitioners.

2) Why have a code?

A code of ethics acts as a specific, identifying feature for a particular professional group, both for the professionals themselves and for the general public. In addition, the need for an explicit code has become more urgent in recent years, as an accelerated pace of social and technological change has produced a sharp increase in the number and complexity of professional situations that demand an ethical response. Finally, the increased speed and frequency of global communications have made the development of a formal statement of shared beliefs and values vital as an agreed point of departure or common language for the profession worldwide.

3) What can a code do?

A code of ethics offers guidance (ideals) for the midwife's professional conduct—the moral 'shoulds' and 'oughts' of life. These 'morals' direct the behaviour of midwives in their relationships with individuals, institutions and the world. The code offers a framework which may enhance midwives' capacity for effective moral decision-making and reflection. It may also provide external agreed criteria by which the appropriateness of a given course of action may be challenged or justified.

4) What can't a code do?

A code of ethics cannot assure ethical practice or "good" decisions in midwifery care; it cannot "tell" one how to make ethical decisions or what to do in every situation; it cannot prevent its misuse; and the code cannot offer specific issues for discussion or resolution. Finally, a code cannot remove from midwives the responsibility and pain of living and acting, at times, in situations of ambiguity or "not knowing", of having no in-built guarantees about what, in a given case, constitutes "right action".

5) What is required for use of a code of ethics?

The main requirements for using a code of ethics as a professional include the commitment to critical thinking (time and moral reasoning); the ability (capacity and willingness) to make decisions; a commitment to being a good moral agent—wanting to do the right thing for the right reasons in caring for others while accepting responsibility for one's own actions and decisions; and an understanding of ethics, of oneself and one's values, and other's values as well.

SUGGESTIONS ON HOW TO USE THE CODE OF ETHICS

The value of a statement of one's professional code of ethics lies in its usefulness in all spheres of professional practice. For the midwife, these spheres of professional practice may include direct care-giving, teaching others, administration and research. The following are suggestions of how the *ICM International Code of Ethics for Midwives* may be used:

In **daily practice,** the Code can be an important tool or reference point (yardstick) when facing decisions on what one "should" do in caring for women and childbearing families. While the statements of the Code may not give absolute direction to your decision making, they can (or the ethical principles they are based upon can) offer a framework for action; e.g., selecting an action that promotes good or prevents harm to women.

Practitioners could use criteria within the code when negotiating with others in an effort to obtain the best outcomes for women and their families. The code can be shared with the public by the posting of printed copies.

In **education,** the midwife teacher has an obligation to help students understand what it means to be a moral agent, to practice ethically, and to identify, understand and accept the dominant values of the profession of midwifery. Teaching methods include a value analysis of each statement of the Code, using the Code in the ethical analysis of critical incidents from midwifery practice, and comparing the basic tenets of the Code for Midwives with those of codes from other professional groups. Critical incident analysis can be a powerful teaching instrument at any level, illuminating practice decisions with the Code's principles as well as with personally identified values.

In **administration,** midwives can use the Code to establish a working environment for ethical practice. Administrators can use the tenets of the Code to define expectations of how midwives will relate to clients, as a framework for ethics discussion groups and for establishing an ethical environment in which employees can function.

In **research,** the Code explicitly defines the ethical approach of the midwives in Statement III.A and Statement IV in its entirety. Researchers, whether midwives or others, should adhere to these basic principles and assure fully informed consent in all research subjects.

ICM 5/1999
Updated 10/2002
Updated 2003

Essential Documents of the National Association of Certified Professional Midwives

CONTENTS

Gender references: To date, most NACPM members are women. For simplicity, this document uses female pronouns to refer to the NACPM member, with the understanding that men may also be NACPM members.

I.   Introduction

The Essential Documents of the NACPM consist of the NACPM Philosophy, the NACPM Scope of Practice, and the Standards for NACPM Practice. They are written for Certified Professional Midwives (CPMs) who are members of the National Association of Certified Professional Midwives.

- They outline the understandings that NACPM members hold about midwifery.
- They identify the nature of responsible midwifery practice.

II. Philosophy and Principles of Practice

NACPM members respect the mystery, sanctity and potential for growth inherent in the experience of pregnancy and birth.

NACPM members understand birth to be a pivotal life event for mother, baby, and family. It is the goal of midwifery care to support and empower the mother and to protect the natural process of birth.

245

NACPM members respect the biological integrity of the processes of pregnancy and birth as aspects of a woman's sexuality.

NACPM members recognize the inseparable and interdependent nature of the mother-baby pair.

NACPM members believe that responsible and ethical midwifery care respects the life of the baby by nurturing and respecting the mother, and, when necessary, counseling and educating her in ways to improve fetal/infant well-being.

NACPM members work as autonomous practitioners, recognizing that this autonomy makes possible a true partnership with the women they serve, and enables them to bring a broad range of skills to the partnership.

NACPM members recognize that decision-making involves a synthesis of knowledge, skills, intuition and clinical judgment.

NACPM members know that the best research demonstrates that out-of-hospital birth is a safe and rational choice for healthy women, and that the out-of-hospital setting provides optimal opportunity for the empowerment of the mother and the support and protection of the normal process of birth.

NACPM members recognize that the mother or baby may on occasion require medical consultation or collaboration.

NACPM members recognize that optimal care of women and babies during pregnancy and birth takes place within a network of relationships with other care providers who can provide service outside the scope of midwifery practice when needed.

III. Scope of Practice for the National Association of Certified Professional Midwives

The NACPM Scope of Practice is founded on the NACPM Philosophy. NACPM members offer expert care, education, counseling and support to women and their families throughout the caregiving partnership, including pregnancy, birth and the postpartum period. NACPM members work with women and families to identify their unique physical, social and emotional needs. They inform, educate and support women in making choices about their care through informed consent. NACPM members provide on-going care throughout pregnancy and continuous, hands-on care during labor, birth and the immediate postpartum period. NACPM members are trained to recognize abnormal or dangerous conditions needing expert help outside their scope. NACPM members each have a plan for consultation and referral when these conditions arise. When needed, they provide emergency care and support for mothers and babies until additional assistance is available. NACPM members may practice and serve women in all settings and have particular expertise in out-of-hospital settings.

IV. The Standards of Practice for NACPM Members

The NACPM member is accountable to the women she serves, to herself, and to the midwifery profession. The NACPM Philosophy and the NACPM Scope of Practice are the foundation for the midwifery practice of the NACPM member. The NACPM Standards of Practice provide a tool for measuring actual practice and appropriate usage of the body of knowledge of midwifery.

Standard One: The NACPM member works in partnership with each woman she serves.
The NACPM member:
- Offers her experience, care, respect, counsel and support to each woman she serves
- Freely shares her midwifery philosophy, professional standards, personal scope of practice and expertise, as well as any limitations imposed upon her practice by local regulatory agencies and state law
- Recognizes that each woman she cares for is responsible for her own health and well-being
- Accepts the right of each woman to make decisions about her general health care and her pregnancy and birthing experience
- Negotiates her role as caregiver with the woman and clearly identifies mutual and individual responsibilities, as well as fees for her services
- Communicates openly and interactively with each woman she serves
- Provides for the social, psychological, physical, emotional, spiritual and cultural needs of each woman
- Does not impose her value system on the woman
- Solicits and respects the woman's input regarding her own state of health
- Respects the importance of others in the woman's life.

Standard Two: Midwifery actions are prioritized to optimize well-being and minimize risk, with attention to the individual needs of each woman and baby.
The NACPM member:
- Supports the natural process of pregnancy and childbirth
- Provides continuous care, when possible, to protect the integrity of the woman's experience and the birth and to bring a broad range of skills and services into each woman's care
- Bases her choices of interventions on empirical and/or research evidence, verifying that the probable benefits outweigh the risks
- Strives to minimize technological interventions

- Demonstrates competency in emergencies and gives priority to potentially life-threatening situations
- Refers the woman or baby to appropriate professionals when either needs care outside her scope of practice or expertise
- Works collaboratively with other health professionals
- Continues to provide supportive care when care is transferred to another provider, if possible, unless the mother declines
- Maintains her own health and well-being to optimize her ability to provide care.

Standard Three: The midwife supports each woman's right to plan her care according to her needs and desires.
The NACPM member:
- Shares all relevant information in language that is understandable to the woman
- Supports the woman in seeking information from a variety of sources to facilitate informed decision-making
- Reviews options with the woman and addresses her questions and concerns
- Respects the woman's right to decline treatments or procedures and properly documents her choices
- Develops and documents a plan for midwifery care together with the woman
- Clearly states and documents when her professional judgment is in conflict with the decision or plans of the woman
- Clearly states and documents when a woman's choices fall outside the NACPM member's legal scope of practice or expertise
- Helps the woman access the type of care she has chosen
- May refuse to provide or continue care and refers the woman to other professionals if she deems the situation or the care requested to be unsafe or unacceptable
- Has the right and responsibility to transfer care in critical situations that she deems to be unsafe.
- She refers the woman to other professionals and remains with the woman until the transfer is complete.

Standard Four: The midwife concludes the caregiving partnership with each woman responsibly.
The NACPM member:
- Continues her partnership with the woman until that partnership is ended at the final postnatal visit or until she or the woman ends the partnership and the midwife documents same

- Ensures that the woman is educated to care for herself and her baby prior to discharge from midwifery care
- Ensures that the woman has had an opportunity to reflect on and discuss her childbirth experience
- Informs the woman and her family of available community support networks and refers appropriately.

Standard Five: The NACPM member collects and records the woman's and baby's health data, problems, decisions and plans comprehensively throughout the caregiving partnership.
The NACPM member:

- Keeps legible records for each woman, beginning at the first formal contact and continuing throughout the caregiving relationship
- Does not share the woman's medical and midwifery records without her permission, except as legally required
- Reviews and updates records at each professional contact with the woman
- Includes the individual nature of each woman's pregnancy in her assessments and documentation
- Uses her assessments as the basis for on-going midwifery care
- Clearly documents her objective findings, decisions and professional actions
- Documents the woman's decisions regarding choices for care, including informed consent or refusal of care
- Makes records and other relevant information accessible and available at all times to the woman and other appropriate persons with the woman's knowledge and consent
- Files legal documents appropriately.

Standard Six: The midwife continuously evaluates and improves her knowledge, skills and practice in her endeavor to provide the best possible care.
The NACPM member:

- Continuously involves the women for whom she provides care in the evaluation of her practice
- Uses feedback from the women she serves to improve her practice
- Collects her practice statistics and uses the data to improve her practice
- Informs each woman she serves of mechanisms for complaints and review, including the NARM peer review and grievance process
- Participates in continuing midwifery education and peer review
- May identify areas for research and may conduct and/or collaborate in research

- Shares research findings and incorporates these into midwifery practice as appropriate
- Knows and understands the history of midwifery in the United States
- Acknowledges that social policies can influence the health of mothers, babies and families; therefore, she acts to influence such policies, as appropriate.

V.   Endorsement of Supportive Statements

NACPM members endorse the **Midwives Model of Care** (© 1996–2004 Midwifery Task Force), the **Mother Friendly Childbirth Initiative** (© 1996 Coalition for Improving Maternity Services) and the **Rights of Childbearing Women** (© 1999 Maternity Center Association, Revised 2004). For the full text of each of these statements, please refer to the following web pages.

Midwives Model of Care (MMOC)
http://cfmidwifery.org/mmoc/define.aspx
Mother Friendly Childbirth Initiative (MFIC)
http://www.motherfriendly.org/MFCI.php
Rights of Childbearing Women
http://www.childbirthconnection.org/

The Code
Standards of Conduct, Performance and Ethics
for Nurses and Midwives

The people in your care must be able to trust you with their health and wellbeing. To justify that trust, you must

- make the care of people your first concern, treating them as individuals and respecting their dignity
- work with others to protect and promote the health and wellbeing of those in your care, their families and carers, and the wider community
- provide a high standard of practice and care at all times
- be open and honest, act with integrity and uphold the reputation of your profession

As a professional, you are personally accountable for actions and omissions in your practice and must always be able to justify your decisions.

You must always act lawfully, whether those laws relate to your professional practice or personal life.

Failure to comply with this Code may bring your fitness to practise into question and endanger your registration.

This Code should be considered together with the Nursing and Midwifery Council's rules, standards, guidance and advice available from www.nmc-uk.org.

Make the care of people your first concern, treating them as individuals and respecting their dignity
Treat people as individuals

- You must treat people as individuals and respect their dignity
- You must not discriminate in any way against those in your care
- You must treat people kindly and considerately
- You must act as an advocate for those in your care, helping them to access relevant health and social care, information and support

Respect people's confidentiality

- You must respect people's right to confidentiality
- You must ensure people are informed about how and why information is shared by those who will be providing their care
- You must disclose information if you believe someone may be at risk of harm, in line with the law of the country in which you are practising

Collaborate with those in your care

- You must listen to the people in your care and respond to their concerns and preferences
- You must support people in caring for themselves to improve and maintain their health
- You must recognise and respect the contribution that people make to their own care and wellbeing
- You must make arrangements to meet people's language and communication needs
- You must share with people, in a way they can understand, the information they want or need to know about their health

Ensure you gain consent

- You must ensure that you gain consent before you begin any treatment or care
- You must respect and support people's rights to accept or decline treatment and care
- You must uphold people's rights to be fully involved in decisions about their care
- You must be aware of the legislation regarding mental capacity, ensuring that people who lack capacity remain at the centre of decision making and are fully safeguarded
- You must be able to demonstrate that you have acted in someone's best interests if you have provided care in an emergency

Maintain clear professional boundaries

- You must refuse any gifts, favours or hospitality that might be interpreted as an attempt to gain preferential treatment
- You must not ask for or accept loans from anyone in your care or anyone close to them
- You must establish and actively maintain clear sexual boundaries at all times with people in your care, their families and carers

Work with others to protect and promote the health and wellbeing of those in your care, their families and carers, and the wider community
Share information with your colleagues

- You must keep your colleagues informed when you are sharing the care of others
- You must work with colleagues to monitor the quality of your work and maintain the safety of those in your care
- You must facilitate students and others to develop their competence

Work effectively as part of a team

- You must work cooperatively within teams and respect the skills, expertise and contributions of your colleagues
- You must be willing to share your skills and experience for the benefit of your colleagues
- You must consult and take advice from colleagues when appropriate
- You must treat your colleagues fairly and without discrimination
- You must make a referral to another practitioner when it is in the best interests of someone in your care

Delegate effectively

- You must establish that anyone you delegate to is able to carry out your instructions
- You must confirm that the outcome of any delegated task meets required standards
- You must make sure that everyone you are responsible for is supervised and supported

Manage risk

- You must act without delay if you believe that you, a colleague or anyone else may be putting someone at risk
- You must inform someone in authority if you experience problems that prevent you working within this Code or other nationally agreed standards
- You must report your concerns in writing if problems in the environment of care are putting people at risk

Provide a high standard of practice and care at all times
Use the best available evidence

- You must deliver care based on the best available evidence or best practice.

- You must ensure any advice you give is evidence based if you are suggesting healthcare products or services
- You must ensure that the use of complementary or alternative therapies is safe and in the best interests of those in your care

Keep your skills and knowledge up to date

- You must have the knowledge and skills for safe and effective practice when working without direct supervision
- You must recognise and work within the limits of your competence
- You must keep your knowledge and skills up to date throughout your working life
- You must take part in appropriate learning and practice activities that maintain and develop your competence and performance

Keep clear and accurate records

- You must keep clear and accurate records of the discussions you have, the assessments you make, the treatment and medicines you give and how effective these have been
- You must complete records as soon as possible after an event has occurred
- You must not tamper with original records in any way
- You must ensure any entries you make in someone's paper records are clearly and legibly signed, dated and timed
- You must ensure any entries you make in someone's electronic records are clearly attributable to you
- You must ensure all records are kept securely

Be open and honest, act with integrity and uphold the reputation of your profession

Act with integrity

- You must demonstrate a personal and professional commitment to equality and diversity
- You must adhere to the laws of the country in which you are practising
- You must inform the NMC if you have been cautioned, charged or found guilty of a criminal offence
- You must inform any employers you work for if your fitness to practise is called into question

Deal with problems

- You must give a constructive and honest response to anyone who complains about the care they have received

- You must not allow someone's complaint to prejudice the care you provide for them
- You must act immediately to put matters right if someone in your care has suffered harm for any reason
- You must explain fully and promptly to the person affected what has happened and the likely effects
- You must cooperate with internal and external investigations

Be impartial

- You must not abuse your privileged position for your own ends
- You must ensure that your professional judgment is not influenced by any commercial considerations

Uphold the reputation of your profession

- You must not use your professional status to promote causes that are not related to health
- You must cooperate with the media only when you can confidently protect the confidential information and dignity of those in your care
- You must uphold the reputation of your profession at all times

Information about indemnity insurance

The NMC recommends that a registered nurse, midwife or specialist community public health nurse, in advising, treating and caring for patients/clients, has professional indemnity insurance. This is in the interests of clients, patients and registrants in the event of claims of professional negligence.

Whilst employers have vicarious liability for the negligent acts and/or omissions of their employees, such cover does not normally extend to activities undertaken outside the registrant's employment. Independent practice would not be covered by vicarious liability. It is the individual registrant's responsibility to establish their insurance status and take appropriate action.

In situations where an employer does not have vicarious liability, the NMC recommends that registrants obtain adequate professional indemnity insurance. If unable to secure professional indemnity insurance, a registrant will need to demonstrate that all their clients/patients are fully informed of this fact and the implications this might have in the event of a claim for professional negligence.

Healthcare professionals have a shared set of values, which find their expression in this Code for nurses and midwives. These values are also reflected in the different codes of each of the UK's healthcare regulators. This Code was approved by the NMC's Council on 6 December 2007 for implementation on 1 May 2008.

Contact
Nursing & Midwifery Council
23 Portland Place
London W1B 1PZ
020 7333 9333
advice@nmc-uk.org
www.nmc-uk.org

Index

Figures and tables are indicated by f and t following the page number.